HEALTH SERVICES IN
THE UNITED STATES

HEALTH SERVICES IN THE UNITED STATES

Second Edition

FLORENCE A. WILSON, M.D.
DUNCAN NEUHAUSER, Ph.D.

BALLINGER PUBLISHING COMPANY
Cambridge, Massachusetts
A Subsidiary of Harper & Row, Publishers, Inc.

International Standard Book Number: 0-88410-713-2

Library of Congress Catalog Card Number: 82-6816

Printed in the United States of America

Library of Congress Cataloging in Publication Data

Wilson, Florence A.
  Health services in the United States.

  Rev. ed. of: Health services in the United States /
Duncan Neuhauser [and] Florence A. Wilson. 1973.
  Includes bibliographies and index.
  1. Medical care — United States. 2. Public health laws — United
States. I. Neuhauser, Duncan. II. Neuhauser, Duncan. Health
services in the United States. III. Title. [DNLM: 1. Delivery of
health care — United States. W 84 AA1 N4h]
  RA395.A3W54 1982   362.1'0973   82-6816
  ISBN 0-88410-713-2   AACR2

To   Elinor T. Neuhauser

CONTENTS

Chapter 7
The Role of State and Local Governments 229

Chapter 8
Voluntary Agencies and Organizations 239

LIST OF FIGURES

LIST OF TABLES

PREFACE

This description of health services in the United States was originally developed for graduate students at the Harvard School of Public Health. The goal of this second edition remains the same as that of the first edition; to provide a concise but reasonably complete summary of major components of health care in this country. To this end, we have extensively revised and updated the work and have added new sections, including a summary of important food and drug laws, and a new chapter on health law and medical ethics.

One might refer to this document as an anatomy of American health services. It stops short of being physiology, that is, how the system works. It stops short of being pathology, that is, how and where the services fail to work. Finally, it does not include the techniques that managers, professionals, or consumers might use to operate, modify, or change health services.

We have attempted to be as objective and dispassionate as possible. However, this is often exceedingly difficult. One can scarcely write a word in this field without it being the potential source of controversy and debate. For example, take the title of this document. We might have referred to the "U.S. Health Services System," but there is an argument as to whether it is a "system" or a "non-system." The social scientists refer to it as a "system," implying that it has a boundary, component parts, and relationships. Some reformers refer to it as a "non-system" implying that it is chaotic and in need of a reorganization along more rational lines. We might have referred to the "U.S. Health Services Industry" but one ideological implication of the word "industry" is that health services are just like the automobile or steel industry and they are or should be all under the control of the market place. We have tried to avoid taking sides but since much of the content has been the focus of political or ideological debates the task is difficult.

A document such as this has other inherent problems. For example, much effort has gone into making it as brief as possible, which leads to the dilemma of what to include and what to exclude and where to place the emphasis. Here our general rule has been to focus on those areas that are most important to the understanding of current issues. Some readers, therefore, may feel that their own occupation or organization has not been covered to the depth they would like. Also, since one of the distinguishing characteristics of American health services is their great diversity and variety, many general descriptive statements may be to some degree misleading or wrong; yet, if every exception were cited this documents would be unduly long. Finally, some of the material will soon be affected by ongoing changes in laws and institutions. Despite these problems, we hope this endeavor will continue to prove useful.

ORGANIZATION OF THE BOOK

The two large divisions of the health care system, *hospitals* and *nursing homes* (institutional care) and *ambulatory care* (noninstitutional care) are described in Chapters 2 and 3. Chapter 4 deals with health professions and occupations. Chapter 5 describes the way care is paid for. Chapter 6 deals with the federal government and is the largest, reflecting the still very important federal role and our objective of assembling in one place a relatively extensive overview of federal legislation. Chapter 7 reviews the role of state and local governments in a more general way, since specific treatment of the various states is beyond the scope of this book. The remaining chapters are concerned with voluntary agencies (Chapter 8); the support industry supplying pharmaceuticals, supplies, equipment, and other services (Chapter 9); a review of approaches to cost and quality control (Chapter 10); and finally, a brief review of some concepts in health law and ethics (Chapter 11).

The selected readings have not been chosen as a systematic or extensive bibliography but rather to complement the book in furthering a general understanding of the organization of health services, to elucidate some historical aspects, and to indicate useful sources of data.

We would like to acknowledge the special contributions of Ruth Chasek, who negotiated the long copy editing process with patience and good humor, and Jane Cerny who assisted valiantly with the index.

Duncan Neuhauser   **Florence A. Wilson**
Cleveland   Boston

HEALTH SERVICES IN THE UNITED STATES

1 INTRODUCTION

The U.S. health care system is highly pluralistic — a complex mix of multiple types of public and private organizations with multiple sources of funding, many points of decisionmaking, and numerous and skilled personnel. It has been undergoing continuous and often rapid change. Its components may be categorized into *institutional care*, rendered to persons who stay for short- or long-term periods in hospitals, nursing homes, and other institutions, and *ambulatory care*, for patients in the community. Interacting with this system are society's values and priorities, in manifestations such as regulation, financing, consumerism, and technology. A complex educational and research system; a collection of manufacturers and suppliers of equipment, drugs, and numerous other items; and many providers of services support and interact with these basic components.

This system has been consuming a steadily rising proportion of national resources, which has now reached 9.4 percent of the gross national product. This has resulted in an increase in cost control activities, particularly through government regulation. A growing concern has been the rapid development and diffusion of new and expensive technology for the diagnosis and treatment of disease. This issue has not only been a feature of the debate concerning costs but has led to many complex legal and ethical questions.

SOME DEFINITIONS

Health. There is no agreed upon definition of health, though a great many have been offered. It is commonly viewed as the absence of illness or disease but many argue that this is too narrow a definition and that concepts such as optimal function and complete well-being should be included. Frequently quoted definitions are that of the World Health Organization: "a state of complete physical, mental and social well-being and not merely the absence of disease or infirmity,"[1] and that of Talcott Parsons: "a state of optimal capacity of an individual for effective performance of the roles and tasks for which he has been socialized."[2] On a more practical level, the Public Health Services' National Center for Health Statistics in one context implicitly defines health in its use of the concept of "disability days" (days on which usual activities cannot be performed) in its Health Interview Survey.

Medical Care. This term has traditionally meant the care of individuals by or under the direction of physicians. It has also often referred (as in "medical care costs" and "medical care organizations") to the aggregate of personal health care including the many non-physician dimensions such as dental care, nursing care, and care by other professionals. In recent years, for complex reasons, partly reflecting dissatisfaction with the restricted scope and physician orientation of "medical," the term "health" has been widely substituted for "medical" and now one sees many references to "health care costs," "health care issues," and the "health care delivery system."[3] Some people, however, object to this substitution, feeling that this inevitably serves to equate "health" with the narrower "medical," whereas health in its broad sense depends in large part on individuals' living habits and on society's willingness to promote a salutary environment.

1. World Health Organization Constitution. Preamble to the Constitution (1946).

2. Talcott Parsons, "Definitions of Health and Illness in the Light of American Values and Social Structure," in E.G. Jaco, ed., *Patients, Physicians and Illness* (Glencoe, Ill.: The Free Press, 1958), p. 176.

3. An interesting discussion of this phenomenon may be found in " 'Hal'—Old Word, New Tasks—Reflections on the Words 'Health' and 'Medical' " by John D. Jago, *Social Science and Medicine* 9 (1975): 1–5.

Public Health. This has traditionally referred to the control of disease in populations as a whole by organized community action, such as through government departments of public health. This has included control of communicable disease and environmental hazards, activities that cannot be carried out in the context of medical care of individuals. A broader concept of public health includes a wide variety of activities for the promotion of health and well-being, ranging from nutrition programs to automobile safety. By extension, the term has come to encompass health-related activities, especially regulation, carried out by public (i.e., government) agencies. Also by extension, it may include health activities carried out *in* the community as opposed to *by* the community. (See "Community Health" below.)

Preventive Medicine. This term also lacks a generally accepted definition. It is most often used to mean disease prevention measures taken in the context of medical care, or as the responsibility of individuals themselves. It may, however, be used much more broadly to include all activities directed toward prevention of disease and disability and the promotion of health whether through traditional public health programs or personal medical care.

Primary prevention generally means the prevention of the occurrence of disease in the first instance, using measures such as environmental sanitation and immunizations, and control of personal habits related to smoking, diet, use of seat belts, and so forth. *Secondary prevention* is the early diagnosis and treatment of disease for cure or limitation of sequelae and complications. *Tertiary prevention* is rehabilitation and the limitation of disability.

Community Health. This term is sometimes substituted for "public health" (as in "community health agency" and "community health nurse"), but is more often used broadly to refer to health-related activities in the community as opposed to hospitals and other institutions. It is often used synonymously with "community medicine" and "ambulatory care."

Need and Demand for Care. *Need for care* usually refers to an expert estimate of the health services a person or population requires. *Demand for care* is defined in two ways: (1) The medical definition is the amount of care that people would use if there were no barriers to use (such as cost or access). (2) The economic definition is the amount of care purchased at a given price. *Realized demand* is the amount of health care actually used. *Unmet need* is the difference between realized demand and need.

SOME STATISTICS [4]

In 1980 the population of the United States was 226,505,000 people, up 11.4 percent from 1970. The median age was 30 years, up from 28 years in 1970. Persons aged 65 and older comprised 11.3 percent of the population, compared with 9.8 percent in 1970. (Demographers note that this trend toward an older population will continue in the coming decades.) Average life expectancy at birth in 1978 was 73.3 years, up from 70.9 in 1970 (and 47.3 in 1900). Infant mortality rate (the number of deaths during the first year of life per 1,000 live births) was 13.8 in 1980, down from 20.0 in 1970 (and 29.2 in 1950).

The major causes of death in the United States are heart disease, cancer, cerebrovascular disease (stroke), and accidents. The respective rates (deaths per 100,000 population) in 1980 were 207.6, 133.8, 45.3, and 44.3. (Total death rate was 883.4.) Half the accidental deaths were from motor vehicle accidents.

Table 1-1 shows national health expenditures for the one-year period ending December 1980, a total of 242.2 billion dollars (9.4 percent of the GNP).

SOURCES OF DATA

A great number of data compilations on various aspects of the health system are produced regularly or intermittently. These include statistics from professional societies and associations, planning agencies, and all levels of government. Important national data sources are the periodic *Health Resources Statistics* publication of the National Center for Health Statistics, and the frequent reports on health expenditures, including Medicare and Medicaid, published by the Health Care Financing Administration. The National Center for Health Statistics

---

4. Sources: Department of Commerce, Bureau of the Census; Monthly Vital Statistics Report, National Center for Health Statistics, September 17, 1980; and the Health Care Financing Administration, Office of Research, Demonstrations, and Statistics.

Table 1-1. National Health Expenditures, Twelve Months through December, 1980.

	Dollars (billions)
Total	247.2
Health Services and Supplies	235.6
Personal health care	217.9
hospital care	99.6
physicians' services	46.6
dentists' services	15.9
other professional services	5.4
drugs and drug sundries	19.2
eyeglasses and appliances	5.1
nursing home care	20.7
other personal health care	5.4
Prepayment/administrative expenses[a]	10.4
Government public health activity	7.3
Research and Construction	11.6
Research	5.4
Construction of medical facilities	6.1
Gross National Product (GNP)	2,626.1
National Health Expenditures as a Percent of GNP	9.4%

a. The amount retained by health insurance organizations for operating expenses, additions to reserves, and profits.

Source: *Health Care Financing Trends*, Health Care Financing Administration, Office of Research, Demonstrations, and Statistics (Winter, 1980).

carries out many surveys and collects and distributes information. Its publication, *Selected National Data Sources for Health Planners*, provides an excellent listing and description of many useful sources of data.

THE SOCIAL WELFARE SYSTEM

Complementing and interacting with the health care system is a complex social welfare system consisting of public welfare departments;[5] children's protective agencies; day-care and foster-care programs;

5. In recent years "public welfare departments" have been widely renamed "departments of social services," "departments of human resources," and so forth.

programs for the elderly; family counseling and service agencies; institutions, homes, shelters; and halfway houses for abandoned and abused children, runaway youth, and destitute adults; and many others. This system is not dealt with as such in this book, but the reader is reminded of its existence and importance.

SELECTED READINGS

Health Care Delivery in the United States, 2nd edition. Steven Jonas and contributors (New York: Springer Publishing Company, 1981).

Introduction to Health Services. Stephen J. Williams and Paul R. Torrens, eds. (New York: John Wiley and Sons, 1980).

Health United States. Published annually by the U.S. Department of Health and Human Services. A compilation of statistics concerning trends in health care and discussions of selected issues.

Medical Care Chartbook, 7th edition. Avedis Donabedian, Solomon J. Axelrod, and Leon Wyszewianski, Department of Medical Care Organization, School of Public Health, the University of Michigan (Washington, D.C.: AUPHA Press, 1980).

2 HOSPITALS AND NURSING HOMES

About 49 percent of the U.S. medical dollar goes to hospitals and nursing homes. Hospitals alone account for 40.2 percent; nursing homes account for the remaining 8.4 percent (1980).

There are no mutually exclusive definitions of hospitals and nursing homes, but they can be distinguished by a number of general attributes. Nursing homes care primarily for patients who need mostly nursing services rather than intensive physician care or diagnostic evaluation. Most nursing home patients are elderly and are relatively long-term residents. The median age of hospital patients is younger and their stays are usually relatively short (however, chronic disease hospital stays are relatively long term). Most hospital patients are admitted from the community while most nursing home patients come from hospitals. Surgery is performed in few if any nursing homes but is an important service in virtually all hospitals (an exception, however, is most private psychiatric hospitals). Many nursing homes have become quite complex and there is now no clear line separating them from hospitals. Many patients are now cared for in nursing homes who a few decades ago would have been in short-term hospitals, chronic disease hospitals, or mental hospitals. Hospitals and nursing homes can be viewed functionally as a continuum of institutions with inpatient beds, ranging from the most highly technological university hospitals to the simplest convalescent and rest

7

homes. They are however sharply distinguished by state licensing definitions and by the government agencies and health insurance organizations that pay for care.

Hospitals can be classified or grouped in a variety of different ways, including type of ownership (government or public, voluntary, and proprietary), type of problem treated (general and specialized hospitals), average length of stay (short term and long term),[1] type of medicine (regular medical and osteopathic), role of education (teaching and nonteaching), and size (usually the number of beds).

HOSPITAL OWNERSHIP

For purposes of understanding the organization of U.S. health services, hospital ownership is a particularly useful way to group hospitals. They can be divided into government-owned and privately owned facilities. Government ownership is at the federal, state, or local level. Private hospitals are subdivided into not-for-profit (voluntary), and for-profit (proprietary) organizations. These types of organizations are summarized in Figure 2-1. Tables 2-1 and 2-2 show hospitals by ownership and numbers of beds.

Federal Government

The following are hospitals that are federally owned.

Department of Defense (DOD): Army, Navy, Air Force. The Department of Defense operates hospitals and clinics whose primary purpose is to provide care for active and retired members of the seven uniformed services (Army, Navy, Marine Corps, Air Force, Coast Guard, Commissioned Corps of the National Oceanic and Atmospheric Administration, and the Commissioned Corps of the Public Health Service) and their dependents. The Civilian Health and Medical Program of the Uniformed Services (CHAMPUS) provides

---

1. Short-term (acute care) and long-term (chronic care) hospitals are distinguished by the average length of stay of inpatients. The American Hospital Association defines a short-term hospital as one in which the average length of stay is less than thirty days or in which 50 percent of all patients are admitted to units where the average length of stay is less than thirty days. Long-term hospitals are often categorized with nursing homes as *long-term care facilities*.

Figure 2-1. Hospitals by Type of Ownership.

Federal Government	Department of Defense	Army Navy Air Force
	Veteran's Administration	
	Department of Health and Human Services	Bureau of Medical Services Indian Health Service Alcohol, Drug Abuse and Mental Health Administration
	Department of Justice — Prisons	
	Department of Transportation — U.S. Coast Guard	
State Government	Long Term (Psychiatric, Chronic disease, Tuberculosis) Short Term (State University Medical School Hospitals, Prison Hospitals)	
Local Government	District County and City	
Voluntary (Not for Profit)	Religious Groups	
	Independent	
	Other	Industrial (Railroad, Lumber, Union) Health Maintenance Organizations (Kaiser-Permanent) Shriners Hospitals Cooperatives (Group Health Cooperative of Puget Sound)
Proprietary (For Profit)	Individual Owner Partnership Corporation	

Table 2-1. Short-Term and Long-Term Hospitals by Ownership.

Ownership	Number
Total	6,998
Federal	361
Psychiatric	24
General and other special	337
Nonfederal	6,627
Psychiatric	527
Not-for-profit	94
Investor owned (for-profit)	146
State and local government	287
Long-term general and nonpsychiatric special	177
Not-for-profit	75
Investor owned (for-profit)	11
State and local government	91
Short-term general and nonpsychiatric special [a]	5,923
Not-for-profit	3,350
Investor owned (for-profit)	727
State and local government	1,846

a. Includes eighty-one hospital units of institutions.

Source: *Hospital Statistics*, 1980 edition. American Hospital Association, Chicago, Data from 1979 Annual Survey.

Table 2-2. Short-Term Nonfederal Hospitals by Ownership and Number of Beds—1979.[a]

Ownership	Number of Beds				
	6-49	50-99	100-299	300-499	Over 500
Not-for-profit	505	686	1,364	540	255
Investor owned (for-profit)	190	190	317	27	3
State and local government	687	587	422	86	64
Total hospitals	1,382	1,463	2,103	653	322

a. Excludes psychiatric hospitals.

Source: *Hospital Statistics*, 1980 edition. American Hospital Association, Chicago, Data from 1979 Annual Survey.

funding for dependents and retired members to receive care in the civilian health care system.

The Army, Navy, and Air Force have their own hospital and health care systems with small clinics and inpatient services on military bases, hospitals serving larger areas, and large medical centers serving regions.

Veterans Administration. The difference between Department of Defense medical care and the Veterans Administration (VA) is that the former serves primarily current members (in addition to retired career personnel) of the armed forces, while the VA serves those who have left the service, largely those with some service connected disability.

In 1980 the Veterans Administration spent $6.2 billion on medical care out of total expenditures of $21.6 billion.[2]

There are 30.1 million living veterans, of whom 26.0 million served during wartime. Potentially, many of these veterans could use VA medical care provided through the 172 hospitals, 226 outpatient clinics, 92 nursing homes and 16 domiciliary facilities distributed throughout the United States. In 1980, 1.25 million inpatients were treated (with an average daily census of 105,085, down 1.6 percent from 1979) and there were 17.9 million outpatient visits (up 4.1 percent).

The VA medical services are divided administratively into twenty-eight Medical Districts and a Central Office in Washington, D.C.

The VA makes a major commitment to medical research and education. It has many affiliation arrangements with educational programs for health professionals, including physicians, nurses, dentists, social workers, and others. One hundred and thirty-seven VA hospitals have affiliation agreements with 104 medical schools, and residencies.

The following types of patients are eligible for care in VA hospitals:

- Those requiring treatment for military service-connected disabilities.

- Those requiring treatment for nonservice-connected conditions who were either discharged from military service for a disability incurred or aggravated in the line of duty, or who have a compensable service-connected disability.

- Other veterans with wartime service who require treatment for nonservice-connected conditions, if they are not able to pay for private hospital care. They must indicate on an affidavit that they

2. Administrator of Veterans Affairs, *Annual Report* (Washington, D.C.: U.S. Government Printing Office, 1980).

are unable to pay for hospital care and include a statement of their assets.

- Military personnel transferred from military hospitals to continue treatment, who are in the process of being discharged from the armed forces.

Since 1977, dependents of living or deceased veterans with total and permanent service-connected disabilities have been entitled to receive care under a program called the Civilian Health and Medical Program of The Veterans Administration (CHAMPVA).

About 70 percent of VA patients are below the poverty level.

Department of Health and Human Services. Agencies of the Department of Health and Human Services (formerly the Department of Health, Education, and Welfare) operate a variety of hospitals:

The Bureau of Medical Services has operated eight Public Health Service (PHS) hospitals and some twenty-six clinics. These facilities are now being turned over to local communities or other government departments. This bureau also operates a long-term care leprosarium in Louisiana.

The Indian Health Service provides care for about half a million American Indians and Alaskan natives. In 1978 it operated 49 hospitals, 83 health centers, about 120 smaller health stations, and school centers in 28 states.

The Alcohol, Drug Abuse and Mental Health Administration cares for neuropsychiatric patients at a clinical research center in Lexington, Kentucky, and jointly operates with the District of Columbia, St. Elizabeths Hospital, a psychiatric hospital for residents of Washington, D.C. and the Virgin Islands.

Other Departments. The *Department of Justice's* Federal Bureau of Prisons provides medical services for prisoners in federal institutions, including a referral medical center for federal prisoners in Springfield, Missouri. The U.S. Coast Guard (*Department of Transportation*) operates two hospitals (in Kodiak, Alaska and New London, Connecticut) in addition to using military hospitals.

State Government

The states operate a wide variety of long-term and short-term hospitals. Every state operates one or more hospitals for the mentally ill and mentally retarded for use by state residents who cannot afford care elsewhere. Admission to mental hospitals can be a voluntary decision on the part of the patient, or an involuntary commitment by a court on the recommendation of a court-appointed board of examiners, which considers petitions from the patient's family and testimony from psychiatrists in a commitment hearing. Involuntary commitments, once frequent, are becoming rarer. Many states also operate one or more chronic disease or tuberculosis hospitals. The number of tuberculosis hospitals has steadily declined in the last thirty years.

A number of states own acute care general hospitals that are controlled by state medical schools. The university hospital of the University of Michigan Medical School in Ann Arbor is an example. States also operate infirmaries connected with state reformatories and prisons, as do some larger counties and cities.

Local Government

District. Hospital districts are similar to school, sanitary, and water districts. They are political subdivisions set up for the purpose of maintaining hospitals, and have the power to tax people in the district. They are governed by officials elected by district residents. This arrangement is widespread for schools, but rare for hospitals and occurs only in some western states, noticeably California.

County and City. County hospitals are run by elected county commissioners or supervisors. Some (usually rural) serve both patients who can pay for private care and those who cannot; these are very much like voluntary hospitals. Other county hospitals (usually urban) and city hospitals were originally established to care for the poor without other sources of care. Most of these are relatively large and are often affiliated with medical schools. Examples are the Cook County Hospital in Chicago, Los Angeles County Hospital, and Boston City Hospital. New York City operates a municipal hospital system of sixteen institutions that includes Bellevue Hospital. Some localities operate long-term hospitals as well as these short-term hospitals.

Voluntary or Nonprofit Hospitals

The words "voluntary" and "nonprofit" in reference to hospitals are used interchangeably.

Religious Groups. A number of religious groups own, operate, or own and operate hospitals. The Roman Catholic Church is foremost of these groups in terms of number of hospitals.

Roman Catholic hospitals are owned and operated by over 100 different sisterhoods, at least one brotherhood (The Alexian Brothers), or by a diocese or archdiocese that is the regional organization of this church. The sisterhoods are religious orders or communities bound together within the Church, self-sufficient, relatively independent, and abiding by the canon laws of the Church. Traditionally, but not always, the Mother Superior (sometimes Mother General or Mother Provincial) of the order acts as president of the hospital board, a sister is administrator, and sisters work in a variety of capacities within the hospital, although they are usually only a small fraction of the hospital's total workforce. In the last two decades there has been an increasing number of lay (in the religious sense of the word) administrators and board members. Traditionally the hospitals of an order were loosely linked together; however some orders, such as the Sisters of Mercy, have centralized specialized management functions in a way that is somewhat similar to large business corporations.

Over a dozen Protestant denominations have been instrumental in founding hospitals. Some continue to direct the operation of their hospitals, for example, the Latter Day Saints (Mormons) and the Salvation Army, while others, such as the Methodists and Lutherans, have allowed their hospitals to become largely independent institutions.

Hospitals are not specifically owned or operated by Jewish religious organizations, but a number of independent voluntary hospitals are supported by the local Jewish community.

Independent Voluntary Hospitals. These nonprofit hospitals were formed as corporations for the sole purpose of providing hospital care to a community. The public spirited citizens who originally created them formed boards of trustees to be responsible for the operation of these hospitals. The trustees usually choose new members to fill vacancies and thus are self-perpetuating boards. Sometimes there is a larger group (called incorporators, the corporation, or the society) from whom the board members are drawn. Sometimes the board is the equivalent of the corporation.

A number of ethnic or nationality groups have founded hospitals. This tendency was much stronger at the beginning of this century when Norwegian, French, Swedish, Black, and other groups founded hospitals. Originally these hospitals largely served these groups, but now they are almost indistinguishable from other independent voluntary hospitals.

Other Types of Voluntary Ownership. A few hospitals are owned by industrial corporations for their employees (railroads, logging), and by unions for their members. Some hospitals are owned by health maintenance organizations (HMOs), notably the hospitals of The Kaiser–Permanente Health Plans in California. A few hospitals are cooperatively owned by the users of their services, such as the Group Health Cooperative of Puget Sound in the state of Washington. The Shriners (The Ancient Arabic Order of the Mystic Shrine of North America, a fraternal organization), own and operate hospitals for crippled children under the age of fourteen who are unable to pay the full costs of their care and who have a possibility of cure or rehabilitation to self-sufficiency.

Proprietary or For-Profit Hospitals

These hospitals have traditionally been owned by one physician (*individual owner*) or a group of physicians (as a *partnership* or *corporation*), who have usually used these hospitals for the care of their own patients.[3]

---

3. Bruce Steinwald and Duncan Neuhauser, "The Role of the Proprietary Hospital," *Journal of Law and Contemporary Problems* (August 1970). Also, Clark V. Havighurst, ed., *Health Care* (New York: Oceana Publications, 1972).

A new development in the last decade has been the growth of investor-owned hospital corporations (*hospital chains, hospital management corporations*). The stock of the larger of these corporations is publicly bought and sold on the stock exchanges. They may own and manage not only hospitals but also nursing homes, health maintenance organizations, clinical laboratories, and such, in the United States and abroad. Some of their recent growth has been in the area of *management contracts*, whereby they contractually undertake to manage hospitals that they do not own. These corporations have central offices and specialized staff and publicly emphasize their managerial expertise. Among the largest of these investor-owned hospital groups or hospital management companies are American Medical International, Hospital Corporation of America, and Humana. The Hospital Corporation of America is the largest, owning or managing over 300 hospitals. (The Whittaker Corporation is an example of a large conglomerate that includes, in addition to its nonhealth activities, a hospital management division). The national association for these companies is the Federation of American Hospitals.

OTHER WAYS TO CLASSIFY HOSPITALS

General and Specialty Hospitals

General hospitals provide care for adult medical and surgical patients and often, but not always, for pediatric and maternity patients. In addition, many other specialized patient services may also be provided, including psychiatric units. In the last twenty years there has been a trend toward closing and consolidating maternity and pediatric services, in part under the pressure of regulatory agencies.

Many *specialty hospitals* have been established to provide care for specific and specialized medical problems. Such hospitals include childrens' (often considered general hospitals for children), maternity, orthopedic, cancer, eye and ear, psychiatric, alcoholism and drug dependency, mental retardation, tuberculosis, and chronic disease.

Medical and Osteopathic Hospitals

In addition to regular medical hospitals, there are voluntary and proprietary hospitals staffed by osteopathic physicians (see p. 71).

There are 204 such hospitals of which 143 are nonprofit voluntary. Osteopathic internships are offered by 102 hospitals and 80 have osteopathic specialty residency training programs.[4] The national association is the *American Osteopathic Association.*

Teaching Hospitals

Although definitions vary, teaching hospitals usually refer to the existence of approved physician residency training programs. A less frequent definition of a teaching hospital is one with an agreement with a medical school to provide clinical experience for medical students. Medical school affiliation may range from direct ownerhsip of the hospital by the medical school to very loosely organized affiliation agreements with otherwise independent hospitals. A third and broadest definition of a teaching hospital is one that provides education and training to any students in the health professions, including nursing students.

In 1980, about 1,372 hospitals offered residency programs. There were about 64,600 residents of whom 18.7 percent were graduates of foreign medical schools.[5] After 1975 the internship was eliminated as the first-year position, and was replaced by the first year of an integrated residency program. (Osteopathic physician training programs have retained the internship.)

Community Hospitals

There is no widely accepted definition of a "community hospital." They are sometimes defined as those serving primarily a local population in contrast to a "referral" hospital that receives many of its patients from a wide area. Community hospitals are sometimes defined as nonteaching hospitals or, more commonly, as nonuniversity hospitals. On the other hand, the American Hospital Association in its statistical reports defines community hospitals as all nonfederal short-term hospitals whose facilities are open to the public.

4. 1981 Directory of the American Osteopathic Hospital Association.

5. "Graduate Medical Education in the United States," *Journal of the American Medical Association* 244 (1980): 2828.

"Tertiary Care" Hospitals

This term has recently been applied to those hospitals, particularly university hospitals that have the most complex diagnostic and therapeutic armamentarium and manage, often on referral from other hospitals, patients with particularly complicated problems.

"Medical Centers"

The term "medical center" has been adopted by many hospitals and hospital groups ranging from single hospitals to complexes of geographically related affiliated institutions, often including a medical school. It implies complexity and special expertise.

Multihospital Arrangements

An increasing number of hospitals are joining together to share ownership and/or services. In 1978 an American Hospital Association survey found that 80 percent of the nation's hospitals shared at least one service. Such arrangements include formal affiliations, as with a medical school; shared or cooperative services, such as group purchasing; consortia for planning or education; contract management; leasing or sharing of property; and corporate ownership and management of more than one hospital. *Multihospital systems* with a single organization owning and managing more than one hospital, include the Veteran's Administration, Catholic orders, Kaiser–Permanente, and the hospital management companies. Over 25 percent of all hospitals are now in some form of multihospital system.

THE GENERAL HOSPITAL: ITS INTERNAL CHARACTERISTICS

The general hospital is described here in considerable detail since it is the most common and familiar type of hospital and accounts for most admissions. The following can be viewed as typical arrangements in a large teaching hospital. Most hospitals have a smaller range of services. It is important to remember that there are endless variations in hospital characteristics.

The governing and legally responsible body of the hospital is the board of trustees (board of governors, board of overseers).[6] The board typically has five to fifteen members, meets monthly, has by-laws, and elects its own officers. It is subdivided into various committees, such as executive, finance, and fund raising. The executive committee typically meets weekly, appoints the administrator, and approves the appointments of physicians and other professionals to the hospital medical staff. The administrator, in turn, appoints department heads and is in charge of the day-to-day operation of the hospital. (In the past superintendent was the common term, then administrator. Currently, titles such as general director, president, or chief executive officer (CEO) are often used.)

The general hospital has several major components. These are the medical staff and its organization, nursing services, medical departments, patient support services, and general administrative and support services.

The Medical Staff (Medical and Dental Staff, Professional Staff)

The medical or professional staff consists primarily of physicians but may also include dentists, podiatrists, psychologists, and other professionals with doctoral degrees. The staff usually has an elected president and/or chief of staff.

An *open staff* is one where any licensed physician may admit his or her private patient to the hospital and care for the patient there. Although this used to be widespread, it is now very rare. A *closed staff* is one where only those physicians whose applications for staff membership have been reviewed and approved by the hospital's governing body (board of trustees) may admit and care for patients. This is now the customary arrangement.

Usually a physician who desires to be on the staff of the hospital submits a written application. This application is reviewed by a credentials' committee of the medical staff. This committee makes an advisory recommendation to the board of trustees, which has the final legal authority to grant staff membership.

---

6. The work of the board of trustees is called *governance*.

Many hospitals have several categories of medical staff, which can include the following:

Active staff: The regular membership.

Associate: Membership for physicians newly appointed to the staff or physicians who may work in the OPD or as research fellows without admitting privileges.

Consulting: Physicians who can consult but not admit.

Courtesy: Physicians who only occasionally use the hospital.

Emeritus: Physicians retired from the active staff.

House staff: Residents (formerly interns and residents).

Honorary: Noted physicians not heavily involved in the hospital.

Usually staff appointments are renewable yearly. In exchange for the privilege of admitting patients to the hospital, active staff physicians are expected to participate in medical staff activities such as committees and teaching. The amount of participation varies substantially with the hospital.

Medical Staff Bylaws.   The *medical staff bylaws* are rules and regulations that govern the physicians of the medical staff. These bylaws are developed by the medical staff and approved by the governing body of the hospital. They vary from hospital to hospital, but generally include reference to the following:

Statement of purpose: Sets forth the purposes of the professional staff organization.

Membership: Qualifications for membership; ethical conduct; terms of appointment; and procedures for appointment, for removal or suspension, and appeals.[7] (Staff appointments for each professional may include a specific *delineation of privileges*, particularly for surgery.

Medical staff organization: Includes categories of membership, organization of clinical departments, election of officers, and procedures for staff meetings (types, frequency, rules of order).

7. It has been established through the courts that professional staff members may not be removed without "due process," as set forth in staff bylaws.

Committees: The composition and responsibilities of the committees through which the medical staff functions are carried out.

Rules and regulations: Detailed policies and procedures governing admission and discharge of patients, medical records, general patient care,[8] and the use of the operating rooms.

The staff usually has an overall elected president and/or chief of staff. The medical staff in all but the smallest hospitals is organizationally divided by major specialty into departments or services such as anesthesiology, family medicine, medicine (internal medicine), obstetrics and gynecology, orthopedic surgery, pathology, pediatrics, radiology, and surgery. Each specialty has a chief of service (or director) and a more or less formally structured organization with meetings, educational programs, and defined policies. There may also be a director of medical education (usually in hospitals without full time chiefs of service) responsible for the residency teaching program.

These positions may be appointed by the governing body or elected by the medical staff or some combination. They may be salaried in full, in part, or not at all. They may have an office in the hospital or may not.

Medical Staff Committees.   Some important examples include:

The *executive committee*, which consists of the chiefs of service, elected members of the staff, and other officers, and is the senior decisionmaking body of the medical staff.

The *joint conference committee*, which includes officers of the medical staff and members of the governing board for the purpose of maintaining communications between board and staff. Not all hospitals have this committee.

The *credentials committee*, which reviews applications for staff membership.

The *utilization review committee*, which reviews patient records to insure that it is necessary for patients to be in the hospital. It may

---

8. These include rules insuring that tissue removed at surgery is sent to the laboratory, the routine physical examination of all patients on admission, the recording of preoperative diagnoses, that surgical patients give written consent to operations, that special cases receive consultations, and many others.

be a separate committee or a part of the *medical audit* committee, which is responsible for reviewing quality of care.

The *tissue committee*, which reviews reports of the examination of surgical specimens. It is presumed to be a check on surgical performance.

The *medical records, infection,* and *pharmacy committees,* which review performance in these areas of the hospital in connection with medical staff activities.

The extent of committees, full-time chiefs of staff, and formalized medical staff rules depends on the size of the hospital. Larger hospitals tend to be more structured and formalized.

Hospital Departments and Services

Hospitals are organized in two different ways simultaneously. The first way is by patients grouped together on patient floors or *nursing units.*[9] The medical specialties with direct care responsibilities are associated with these groups of inpatient beds. For example, a pediatric service will have beds in a designated part of the hospital (nursing unit), a chief of pediatrics, and pediatric staff responsible for patients on this unit. Other personnel such as social workers may also be assigned to the service.

In addition to the regular patient floors there may be various special care units such as intensive care (ICU), coronary care (CCU), renal dialysis, and burn care. Some hospitals have established separately licensed extended care units for patients requiring supervised convalescence or active rehabilitation (see section on nursing homes, page 36).

The second way the hospital is organized is by functional departments that cut across the patient care units; these include nursing, ancillary, administrative, and support departments or services. There is no clear and consistently used difference in the words "service" and "department." Several services or departments may be grouped together in *divisions.* An example of a hospital table of organization is shown in Figure 2–2. There are probably as many variations in organization as there are hospitals with respect to services offered, how

---

9. These units in the past were often called "wards," referring to the prevalent large open units containing several or many patient beds. These have largely been replaced by two to four bed "semiprivate" rooms.

Figure 2-2. A 300 Bed General Hospital.

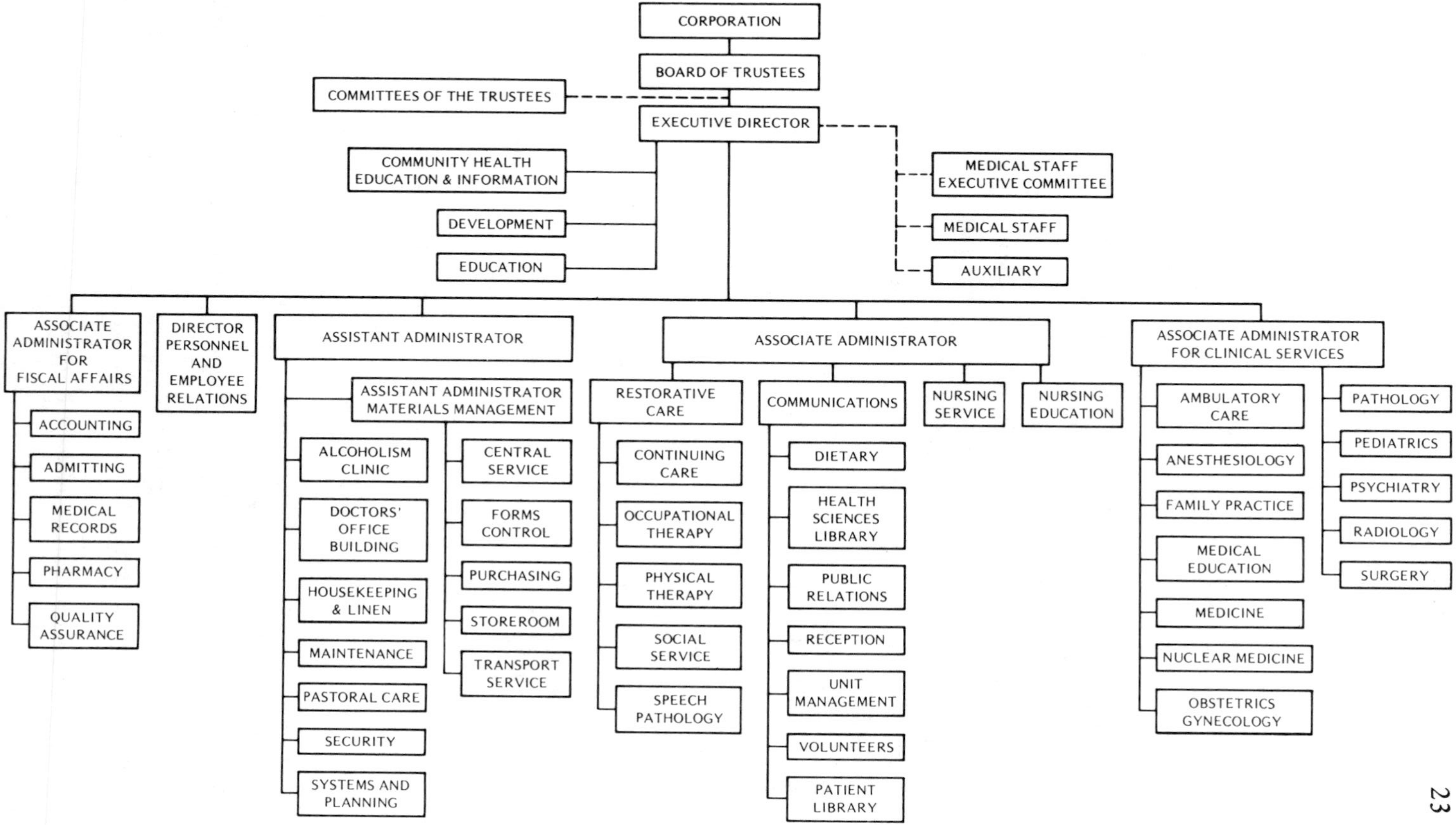

they are grouped together, and their physical location within the hospital.[10]

Nursing Services (Department of Nursing, Division of Nursing). The nursing department is the single largest component of the hospital. It includes a *director of nursing*, responsible for the whole department; and *nursing supervisors*, responsible for several nursing units, each of which is run by a *head nurse* who directs a group of nursing personnel, including professional nurses (RNs), practical nurses (LPNs), nursing aides, and orderlies. There also may be student nurses gaining practical experience. There is usually a *ward clerk* who copes with the paperwork at the nursing station, where the medical records and medications are kept, and a *unit manager* who carries out a variety of managerial activities, including the maintenance of equipment and supplies, thereby freeing nursing personnel for the care of patients.

Nursing is responsible for the care of patients on a twenty-four hour basis. In order to maintain twenty-four hour coverage, seven days a week, there are three daily nursing shifts: usually a day shift, 7 A.M. to 3 P.M.; an evening shift, 3 P.M. to 11 P.M.; and a night shift, 11 P.M. to 7 A.M.

Other nursing service functions may include the general supervision of the *operating suite*, which consists of *operating rooms* (ORs), storage, and associated space such as the *recovery room*, where patients stay immediately after the operation under close supervision before returning to their bed on the nursing unit. For obstetrical patients there are *labor rooms, delivery rooms*, and a *newborn nursery* with bassinets for the newborn babies. Maintenance of special cleanliness is vital in all these units and elaborate precautions are taken to prevent infections.

Nursing education may include a hospital school of nursing (a *diploma school*) and *inservice nursing education*. Hospitals that do not have a school of nursing may provide clinical education for nursing students from junior colleges, colleges, or universities for professional nurses (RNs), and from schools for practical nurses (LPNs).

Medical Departments. These are the medical specialty departments, such as medicine, surgery, pediatrics, with direct primary patient care

---

10. For descriptions of types of personnel and their education, see the chapter on health manpower (Chapter 4).

responsibility and associated with designated patient care floors or units. There are usually subdepartments (subspecialties) such as cardiology, hematology, and neurology (medicine), and neurosurgery and thoracic surgery. There may be associated research laboratories and personnel. There is often a *dental department* with dental specialties.

Ancillary Medical Departments. These are medical specialty departments whose physicians and other personnel provide direct patient services including diagnostic and therapeutic procedures but do not in general have primary ongoing responsibility for patients. All hospitals have departments of anesthesiology, pathology (laboratories), and radiology. Some have departments of *physical medicine (rehabilitation medicine)*.[11]

Anesthesiology. This is a specialty of medicine concerned with the administration of local and general anesthetics, primarily in connection with surgery. This department may include *anesthesiologists* (who are physicians) and *nurse-anesthetists*, both of whom administer anesthesia. *Respiratory (inhalation) therapy* may be included within this department. The postoperative recovery room is frequently the responsibility of this department.

Radiology. This department is directed by a *radiologist* (who is a physician), using x-rays (or Roentgen rays) for the diagnosis (*diagnostic radiology*) and treatment (*radiation therapy*) of disease. The department of nuclear medicine is sometimes associated with the radiology department. *Nuclear medicine* uses radioactive isotopes for the diagnosis and treatment of disease.

The radiology department requires a substantial amount of costly equipment and a physical space constructed so as to minimize the hazard of unwanted radiation exposure.

Pathology (Laboratories). The hospital laboratories perform examination and analysis of tests on human tissue, fluids, and excre-

---

11. Hospital-based physicians working full time within the hospital, particularly anesthesiologists, pathologists, radiologists, and psychiatrists, may be paid in a number of different ways, including: (1) a salary from the hospital; (2) directly billing patients for their services; (3) a percentage of their department's gross income; (4) a percentage of their department's net income; or (5) a combination of these.

tions to aid in the diagnosis and treatment of patients. They are usually under the supervision of the hospital's pathologist-in-chief and, in a very large hospital, may include as many as sixty different subdepartments that do special types of analysis and related research. Major subcomponents include:

The clinical laboratory (clinical pathology), which performs tests on blood, urine, bacteria, parasites, and so forth. It includes *hematology* (the study of blood), *biochemistry* (including the use of automatic analyzers), *bacteriology* (growth and identification of bacteria), *histology* (preparation of tissue removed during surgery), and *cytology* (preparation of body fluids to detect cell changes, such as those related to cancer).

The blood bank maintains a supply of blood and blood derivatives such as plasma, for use in the hospital. In large hospitals there may be *organ banks* (e.g., an eye bank) that maintain a supply of human tissue and bone for replacement in other patients.

The anatomical laboratory examines tissue both grossly (gross anatomy) and with the microscope (microscopic anatomy). *Autopsies* are performed here to determine the causes of death, and a *morgue* for the dead is maintained.

Physical Medicine (Physical and Rehabilitative Medicine). Physical medicine (physiatry) is a specialty of medicine involved with the diagnosis and treatment of the disabled, convalescent, and physically handicapped patient, using such things as heat, special exercises, and hydrotherapy. *Physical therapists* work with the *physiatrist* (a physician) in these tasks.

This department may also include *occupational therapy* and *speech therapy.* Occupational therapists help handicapped patients learn job-related skills and activities of daily living. Speech therapists help patients overcome speech problems.

In a few hospitals, the physical medicine and rehabilitation department may have designated beds to which patients may be admitted or transferred from other services.[12] In hospitals without a medical department of physical medicine there is generally a physiotherapy

---

12. There also exist *rehabilitation centers*, separately licensed institutions to which patients are admitted for rehabilitation treatment.

department whose personnel evaluate and treat patients upon prescription of their physicians.

Patient Support Services.   There are a number of important professional services that supplement the medical care of patients.

The Pharmacy.   This service usually purchases drugs and medications, maintains its supply, fills requisitions for the nursing *floor stock*, and fills prescriptions for individual patients. It is run by the chief pharmacist; a drug and therapeutics committee provides a link with the medical staff. The hospital may maintain a *formulary*, which lists drugs that the medical staff finds acceptable for use in the hospital. It may list drugs by their generic names and permit the pharmacist to substitute between clinically similar drugs. This lowers the drug inventory and lowers the cost of drugs by allowing the pharmacist to purchase in bulk and to use low-cost generic name drugs.

Social Service (Medical and Psychiatric Social Work).   This service focuses on the social, economic, and environmental factors influencing the patient's condition. Knowledge of community resources is used to reduce the environmental and emotional obstacles to recovery, including financial support, posthospital care, and working with the patient's family. Social service often works very closely with psychiatry (psychiatric social work).

Discharge planning.   A special *discharge planning unit* now exists in most hospitals. It may be a part of the social service department, or be a separate unit responsible to administration. The staff of the unit, often including both nurses and social workers, assists patients and families with planning posthospital care, particularly where this involves referral to a home care program or arrangements for a nursing home.

Dietary Services.   This department includes the kitchen, inpatient food service, cafeteria, food storage and purchasing, catering for special events, educational programs for dieticians, and a special diet kitchen. A substantial number of patients may be on special diets (salt free, low fat, etc.). The dietary services department may be headed by a *chief dietician*, a *food service manager*, or both. The education of dieticians emphasizes nutrition, the preparation of special diets, and the relationship between food and health. The background and education of food service managers emphasize the production and management aspects of food preparation.

Chaplaincy Service. This service provides pastoral care and religious counseling for patients.

General Administration and Support Services. These departments are responsible for the overall functioning of the hospital.

Administration. The administrator (various titles are used) and associated general administrative personnel (associate and assistant administrators) have the day-to-day responsibility for managing the hospital. Among these there may be included persons with special competence in systems analysis (industrial engineering), law, and planning. In addition there are specialized administrative departments such as financial affairs, public relations, and personnel, which are among those described below.

The Financial Affairs Office, Comptroller's Office. This office produces patient bills, collects money from patients and third-party payers (accounts receivable), and pays bills (accounts payable). It maintains financial records, prepares budgets and cost reports for the hospital, and does the payroll for hospital employees.

The Public Relations Department. This department provides information about the hospital to the patients, the public, and the press. Sometimes associated with this department (or in a separate department) are *patient representatives* (*patient advocates*), who are responsible for handling patients' problems related to their hospital stay. *Fund raising* may be a temporary or permanent unit that solicits gifts and donations to the hospital, often in connection with the construction of new facilities.

Admissions (Admitting Office, Admitting Department). This department schedules patients for admission, and keeps a waiting list and a list of empty beds. The admissions personnel assigns patients to beds; collects the initial nonmedical information, including financial information; and notifies other parts of the hospital of the admission.

Medical Records Department. This department maintains, stores, and retrieves patient records and associated patient care statistics. A numbering system is maintained for patient records and an index of patient names and record numbers is maintained to facilitate retrieval. The records must be complete, signed by the doctor(s) responsible for the patient, and kept confidential so that only authorized personnel may see them. The *medical records administrator* in charge of this department supervises the file clerks, medical transcriptionists, and medical record technicians working in the department.

The *medical record* is the written record of the patient's progress. Each patient seen in a hospital and in a doctor's private office has a record. When the patient is in the hospital, this record is kept at the nursing station and is also referred to as the *patient's chart.* When the patient is not in the hospital, the chart becomes the medical record and is stored in the medical records department.

The medical record contains several sections including an *admissions form* (patient's age, sex, address, attending physician and admission diagnosis); *initial evaluation* (medical history, physical examination, and plan for treatment); *nursing care plan* and *nurses' notes*; daily record of temperature, pulse, and respirations (TPR), weight, and medications; physician's *progress notes*, including special procedures; *laboratory and x-ray reports*, and other special reports including detailed operative notes; and a *discharge note* with a summary of the hospitalization, discharge diagnosis, and plan of future treatment.[13]

Some hospitals are experimenting with computerization of medical records.

Medical Library. The medical library maintains scientific books and journals for the use of the professional staff and students.

---

13. The *problem-oriented medical record*, developed by Dr. Lawrence L. Weed, is a reorganization of professional recording in the medical record. It changes the focus from the admitting diagnosis to a numbered list of all the patient's problems. Progress toward the resolution of each of these problems is pursued as the focus of the patient's record. Dr. Weed argues that this form of record is better particularly for teaching students and compels attention to the full range of the patient's problems. See Lawrence L. Weed, "Medical Records That Guide and Teach," *New England Journal of Medicine* 278 (1968): 593–600, 652–657; also Stephen E. Goldfinger, "The Problem-Oriented Record: A Critique from a Believer," *New England Journal of Medicine* (1973): 288–606.

Personnel Department. This department recruits, interviews, and screens applicants for hospital positions, and maintains salary scales and employee benefits. It keeps records of present and past hospital employees, orients new employees to the hospital, and maintains a position control system so that the complement of hospital jobs cannot be increased without approval of the administration. Personnel may perform many other functions, including labor relations, particularly if hospital personnel are unionized.

Purchasing and Stores. This is the department responsible for ordering supplies and equipment. It receives, stores, and delivers these items to the part of the hospital where they will be used. Competitive bids are sent out for high cost items and the hospital may participate with other hospitals in the area in a *joint purchasing program*, which can save money by purchasing in large volume.

Communications. This includes the *messenger and transport service*, which delivers mail, supplies, and sometimes moves patients; and the *telephone switchboard*, which receives incoming calls and maintains a paging system for reaching physicians in the hospital. A *patient information service* maintains a list of hospitalized patients, their location, and general condition.

Some hospitals contract for services such as laundry, data processing, housekeeping, dietary, and others, with outside companies, or perform these services jointly with other hospitals (*shared services*). This is a rapidly increasing practice.

Central Supply (also called Central Medical and Surgical Supply, and Central Sterile Supply). This department washes, packages, and sterilizes (autoclaves) equipment, instruments, gowns, dressings, and other items, primarily for the operating rooms, but also for all parts of the hospital where sterile materials are required. Central Supply may also be responsible for distribution of intravenous solutions (IV fluids).

Housekeeping. This department is responsible for maintaining a clean hospital. This can include making beds; washing floors, walls, and windows; and trash collection. *Laundry and Linen* is responsible for laundry and repair of linen, gowns, uniforms, and other laundry.

Maintenance and Plant. This department is responsible for painting, repairs, carpentry, plumbing, the steam plant, electricity, air conditioning, elevators, fire alarm systems, emergency power sources, and so forth. There may be personnel assigned to maintain the hospital's *grounds* (ground crew), and to run areas such as the *parking lot* and *print shop.*

Security. This department is responsible for the physical security of the hospital plant, patients, and personnel.

Volunteers (Auxiliaries). These are public-spirited citizens who donate their time to work for the hospital. They may help in a variety of tasks from escorting patients to running a gift shop, coffee shop, or thrift shop (which sells second-hand clothing, books, furniture, etc., and is located outside the hospital), with the proceeds donated to the hospital. Teenage girls who volunteer are often called *candy stripers*, because of the color of the uniforms they wear.

Ambulatory Services

Most hospitals provide services to other than inpatients. Traditionally these have been outpatient and emergency services but home care programs are now often included. These may be organized in a separate department or division of ambulatory services or may be separate departments.

Outpatient Department (OPD). This department provides care for the nonemergency ambulatory patient. It may be divided into numerous specialty clinics each with its nursing and clerical personnel. Physicians include various combinations of regular medical staff and house staff. Other professionals may include dentists, podiatrists, psychologists, and social workers. The department may include satellite clinics and community health centers operating under the hospital's license.

Emergency Service [Emergency Room (ER), Emergency Department (ED), Emergency Ward (EW)]. This department provides immediate care around the clock for acutely ill patients although many of the patients using this service may not be acutely ill. Nurses, clerks, and other personnel are assigned to this service. Physician care is often by house staff with various specialists available for consultation and supervision. Increasingly, there is a full-time physician director. There are a growing number of physicians who specialize in emergency medicine, some of whom may contract with hospitals (singly or in groups) for provision of services. In smaller hospitals staffing may be by members of the regular medical staff in rotation. The hospital also may have an ambulance service with specially trained *emergency medical technicians* (EMTs). In many regions, emergency rooms and ambulances are being coordinated in *emergency medical systems* that may include centralized ambulance dispatching procedures and the categorization of emergency departments according to their capacity for handling certain types of emergency care. Some departments, for example, may be designated as *trauma centers.*

Many emergency rooms incorporate or are affiliated with *poison control centers*, which offer immediate telephone advice and referral concerning poisoning.

Home Care.   There may be a hospital-based home care program that provides or coordinates care in patients' homes by physicians, nurses, social workers, and physical therapists. Various types of supplies and equipment may be supplied or arranged for.

Technology

Most of the steadily growing volume of complex medical technology is found in hospitals. This includes x-ray, surgical, and laboratory equipment, and electronic patient monitoring devices. Among the most complex and expensive (and thus subject to the interest of regulatory agencies concerned with cost control) are computerized tomography (CT) x-ray scanners and special radiation therapy equipment (such as cobalt therapy).

Technology has long been a part of medical care. Examples are the *electrocardiogram* (ECG, EKG), which measures electrical impulses from the heart, and the *electroencephalogram* (EEG), which measures electrical brain waves. New electronic techniques, including computers, have enhanced traditional technology—for example, the remote EKG monitoring of ambulatory patients. A rapidly developing new diagnostic technique is ultrasonography—the use of sound waves to examine parts of the body. Echocardiography uses this technique for specialized examination of the heart.

Life support technology, such as respirators, has led to many ethical issues related to the prolongation of life.

Hospital Statistics

The following are frequently used hospital statistics.

Patient Days (Patient Bed Days). The total number of inpatient days of care given in a specified time period. For example, if there were 50 patients in the hospital for each day for 10 days this would be 500 patient days for this time period.

Hospital Beds. The average number of beds, cribs, and pediatric bassinets (excluding bassinets for newborn babies) regularly maintained (set up and staffed for use) for inpatients during a period of time, usually a year.

Bassinets. The bassinets, incubators, and isolators for newborn babies in a nursery.

Admissions. The number of patients accepted for inpatient service in a period of time (excluding births).

Discharges and Deaths. The number of inpatients leaving the hospital in a period of time. This usually excludes newborn babies.

Census (Average Daily Census). The number of inpatients receiving care on an average day (excluding newborns). This is usually calculated by counting the number of patients in the hospital every midnight (*midnight census*).

Occupancy. The ratio of census to beds, usually as a percentage of beds in use.

Average Length of Stay (ALOS). Average stay, in days, of inpatients in a given time period. This can be calculated by dividing the number of patient days by either the number of admissions or the number of discharges and deaths.

Available Bed Days. The average number of beds available for use times the number of days in a given time period. Thus, a 100-bed hospital would have 36,500 available bed days per year.

Staffing Ratio. The total number of hospital employees (full-time equivalents) divided by the average daily census.

Per Diem Cost, Cost per Patient Day. The cost of running the hospital divided by the number of patient days in that time period. Various adjustments or corrections in the cost figures are sometimes made in order to compare hospitals.

Waiting List. An ordered list of patients awaiting admission to the hospital.

Hospital Service Charge (Per Diem Charge). The basic price per day for inpatient care, usually including food, basic nursing care, administrative overhead, use of the facility: those services used by all patients. *Ancillary charges* are for special diagnostic and treatment services, such as lab tests, x-rays, and operating rooms.

Case Mix. The distribution of types of cases cared for in a hospital. The words "case" and "patient" are used interchangeably.

Other Concepts and Terminology

Types of Accommodation. This distinction refers to the type of room the patient occupies in the hospital.

A *private patient* occupies a room alone.

A *semiprivate patient* usually occupies a room with one to three other people (or beds).

A *ward patient* occupies a room with four or more other people (or beds). Although increasingly uncommon, wards are still found in older hospitals.

Private and *ward* also refer to different physician–patient arrangements. Private patients have their own physician whom they pay for services rendered. Ward (or "service") patients are cared for by the residents who are supervised by staff physicians.

Emergency Admission, Emergency Surgery. Cases that must be cared for immediately, in contrast to an *elective admission* (elective surgery), which may be delayed without harm to the patient.

Rounds. "To make rounds" constitutes a physician's visit to the bedsides of his hospitalized patients to note their progress. *Ward rounds (teaching rounds)* are the teaching physician's bedside review of patients for the purpose of supervising and instructing house staff and medical students (*bedside teaching*). *Grand rounds* is the (usually) weekly auditorium conference with description, review, and discussion of a patient (*case presentation*) for the medical staff for continuing education.

Clinicopathological Conference (CPC). A detailed case history is described and an expert, who may or may not be from the medical staff, discusses the case and makes a diagnosis. Then the pathologist reports the findings and diagnosis based on tissue examination.

Progressive Patient Care (PPC). This is a way of dividing hospital patient services according to the severity of illness and the amount of care used by the patients. Hospitals have used all, part, or none of this system. Patient care levels, starting with the most intensive, are:

Intensive care (Intensive Care Unit, ICU), for severely ill patients needing a great deal of nursing care and close supervision. The severity of illness is similar in coronary care units (CCUs), which treat patients with heart attacks.

Intermediate care, for moderately ill patients.

Self-care, for inpatients who can walk about, use a central dining area, and who can cope with activities of daily living.

Long-term care (*Extended Care Unit*), for patients who require long-term care.

Home care is the organized provision of care in the patient's home by nurses, therapists, social workers, physicians, and others.

NURSING HOMES

Prior to 1930 there were very few nursing homes. The Social Security Act of 1935, by making money available to elderly beneficiaries, encouraged the growth of proprietary boarding and nursing homes and the decline of public "poor houses" then serving the indigent aged. Medicare and Medicaid provided further impetus to the growth of nursing homes.

Today, almost one in twenty Americans over sixty-five live in long-term care institutions, mostly nursing homes. Care is provided by a variable mix of registered nurses, licensed practical nurses, and nursing aides (nursing assistants), with the latter category by far predominating.

Types of Nursing Homes

There is no agreed upon set of definitions for the various types of nursing homes. Terminology and criteria vary considerably within the federal government and among the states, with classification generally based on the concept of *levels of care*.

National Center for Health Statistics Classification. The National Center for Health Statistics classifies nursing homes (for purposes of the Master Facility Inventory) as follows: [14]

Nursing Care Home. This is a facility whose primary function is nursing care. One or more full-time registered nurses or licensed practical nurses are employed. This definition encompasses all *skilled nursing facilities* and most *intermediate care facilities* defined below.

Personal Care Home with Nursing. This is a facility whose primary function is personal care but that provides some nursing care. Registered professional or licensed practical nursing staff may or may not be employed. Personal care includes administration of treat-

---

14. National Center for Health Statistics, *The National Nursing Home Survey, 1977 Summary for the United States* (Department of Health, Education, and Welfare, July 1979). The above definitions are abbreviated.

ment or medications; and help with bathing, dressing, eating, and ambulation.

Personal Care Home. This is a facility whose primary function is personal care (and in which no resident received nursing care during the week prior to the National Center for Health Statistics' survey). Registered professional or licensed practical nurses may or may not be employed.

Domiciliary Care Home. This is a facility whose primary function is domiciliary care but that also provides some personal care.

This classification encompasses as "nursing homes" all facilities that provide services in addition to room and board. It includes free-standing facilities and units of institutions such as hospitals and retirement centers. The total number of such homes in 1977 was 18,900 with a total of 1,402,400 beds. By far, the majority (14,500) were proprietary and only 900 had more than 200 beds. (See Table 2-3.)

Medicare and Medicaid Classification. For purposes of the Medicare and Medicaid programs the federal government defines nursing homes eligible for reimbursement as *skilled nursing facilities* or *intermediate care facilities.* They are defined in terms of "conditions for participation" (Medicare) or "standards for payment" (Medicaid) that must be met in order for facilities to be certified to receive payment under these programs.

Skilled Nursing Facility (SNF). These facilities must, among other requirements, provide twenty-four-hour nursing services, including at least one registered nurse on each day shift. Emphasis is on restorative nursing care and rehabilitation, with the availability of physical, speech, and occupational therapy.

Medicare will pay for up to 100 days of care in a skilled nursing facility if:

- The patient has spent at least 3 consecutive days in a hospital and is admitted to SNF within 30 days after discharge
- The patient's physician finds that further care is needed for the illness for which the patient had been hospitalized and

Table 2-3. Number and Percent Distribution of Nursing Homes and Beds by Selected Nursing Home Characteristics; United States, 1977.

Nursing Home Characteristic	Nursing Homes		Beds	
	Number	Percent Distribution	Number	Percent Distribution
All nursing homes	18,900	100.0	1,402,400	100.0
Ownership				
Proprietary	14,500	76.8	971,200	69.3
Voluntary nonprofit	3,400	17.7	295,600	21.1
Government	1,000	5.5	135,700	9.7
Certification				
Skilled nursing facility only	3,600	19.2	294,000	21.0
Medicare and Medicaid	2,100	11.3	204,500	14.6
Medicare	700	3.7	27,000	1.9
Medicaid	800	4.2	62,600	4.5
Skilled nursing facility and intermediate care facility	4,600	24.2	549,400	39.2
Medicare SNF and Medicaid SNF and ICF	2,300	12.3	319,500	22.8
Medicaid SNF and ICF	2,100	10.8	218,700	15.6
Medicare SNF and Medicaid ICF	200	1.1	11,300	.8
Intermediate care facility only	6,000	31.6	391,600	27.9
Not certified	4,700	25.0	167,400	11.9
Bed Size				
Less than 50 beds	8,000	42.3	182,900	13.0
50-99 beds	5,800	30.8	417,800	29.8
100-199 beds	4,200	22.3	546,400	39.0
200 beds or more	900	4.6	255,400	18.2

Note: Figures may not add to totals due to rounding.

Source: 1977 National Nursing Home Survey. National Center for Health Statistics Department of Health and Human Services, 1979.

- Skilled nursing care and rehabilitative services are required by the patient on a daily basis.

If the patient qualifies, Medicare will pay for the first 20 days and for part of the next 80 days. The states include care in skilled nursing facilities in their Medicaid programs with the extent varying considerably from state to state.

Under the original Medicare legislation (1965) SNFs eligible to participate in Medicare were termed *extended care facilities* with the intention of defining a category of care in between a hospital and a skilled nursing home. This reflected the intent of Congress to provide for a period of posthospital care distinct from long-term nursing home care. The term, however, was abandoned under the 1972 amendments although a posthospital nursing home stay is still an "extended care benefit" under Medicare.

Intermediate Care Facility (ICF). These facilities must, among other requirements, have a supervising registered nurse or licensed practical nurse full time on each day shift; a practical nurse must consult with a registered nurse no less than four hours each week. Rehabilitation services by qualified therapists or assistants must be available. Intermediate care facilities provide services to persons who do not require hospital or skilled nursing facility care but whose mental or physical condition requires services above the level of room and board. Intermediate care services are included to some degree in all state Medicaid programs. Medicare does not cover intermediate facility care.

Skilled and intermediate care facilities are not necessarily separate entities. A given facility may be certified as a skilled nursing facility only, as both a skilled and intermediate facility (with specific floors or units being so designated), or as an intermediate facility only. (Table 2-4.)

Many religion-affiliated homes for the aged have been certified as skilled nursing or intermediate care facilities. This has in some instances led to the transfer of patients from these facilities to levels of care not available at the original home.

The general issue of patient transfers among different levels of care as their condition or reimbursement status changes, has been of concern to patients' rights groups and has led, in some states, to the establishment of specific procedures for hearings and appeals.

State Classification. The states may define types of nursing homes under their licensing laws. For example, New York State classifies facilities as *skilled nursing facilities*, *health related facilities* (generally equivalent to intermediate care facilities), and *domiciliary care facilities*. Massachusetts defines three categories of nursing homes:

Skilled Nursing Care Facilities provide "continuous skilled nursing care and meaningful availability of restorative services and other therapeutic services for patients who show potential for improvement or restoration to a stabilized condition or who have a deteriorating condition requiring skilled care." Nursing personnel requirements include a full-time director of nurses, and a full-time nursing supervisor on the day shift five days a week in facilities with more than one unit, and a charge nurse (an RN or LPN) each day, all shifts.

Supportive Nursing Care Facilities (Intermediate Care Facilities) provide "routine nursing services and periodic availability of skilled nursing, restorative and other therapeutic services for patients whose condition is stabilized and who need only supportive nursing care, supervision and observation." Nursing personnel requirements include a full-time supervisor of nurses during the day shift, five days a week; a charge nurse during the day and evening shifts each day for each unit; and a responsible nurse's aide during night shifts.

Resident Care Facilities provide "protective supervision for residents who do not routinely require nursing or other medically related services." A responsible person is to be on the premises at all times.

Other Facilities

Adult Homes (Boarding homes). There has been a rapid increase in the number of these facilities since the deinstitutionalization of many mental hospital patients and the advent of the federal Supplemental Security Income (SSI) program in 1972, which provides cash benefits to elderly and disabled poor persons. They are usually proprietary institutions and often are converted hotels. Many elderly persons without family resources reside in these homes either as a preferred alternative to a nursing home or because their needs have been deemed not to require the Medicare/Medicaid funded skilled or intermediate care facilities.

Halfway Houses. These are homes usually developed under public or nonprofit auspices where mentally or physically handicapped persons share living facilities, usually under the general supervision of counselors.

Congregate Housing. This refers to housing for the elderly in which residents share some facilities, often including meal services, and where special social services are available. Persons in such housing have been made eligible for additional SSI benefits.

Regulation

Nursing homes are *licensed* by the state; many and varied regulatory activities are carried out under the licensing laws, activities particularly directed to safety and quality. Increasingly, patients' rights statutes are also being enacted. Homes are *certified* for participation in the Medicare and Medicaid programs. This is generally done by state health departments, who determine compliance with federal standards and requirements. A voluntary program of *accreditation* of long-term care facilities (including nursing homes) is carried out by the Joint Commission on Accreditation of Hospitals.

Nursing home administrators are licensed in all states. Such licensure was mandated in 1972 as a condition of nursing home participation in Medicare. Boarding homes, largely unregulated in the past, are beginning to come under state licensing laws.

Associations

American Health Care Association[15] : Profit and nonprofit homes.
American Association of Homes for the Aged : Nonprofit homes.
National Council of Health Care Services : Corporate nursing home chains.

---

15. Formerly American Nursing Home Association.

SELECTED READINGS

Principles of Hospital Administration, 2nd edition. John R. McGibony (New York: G. P. Putnam's Sons, 1976).

Hospitals: What They Are and How They Work. I. Donald Snook (Rockville, MD: Aspen Publications, 1981).

The Medical Staff in the Modern Hospital. C. Wesley Eisele, ed. (New York: McGraw–Hill, 1967).

Investor-Owned Hospitals and Their Role in the Changing U.S. Health Care System. The Research Staff of F&S Press with Ekaterini Siafaca (New York: F&S Press, 1981).

Cumulative Guide to Hospital Literature. American Hospital Association, Chicago, quarterly.

Hospital Statistics. American Hospital Association, yearly.

Glossary of Hospital Terms, 4th edition. American Medical Record Association (Chicago: The association, 1979).

Directories

American Hospital Association Guide to the Health Care Field. American Hospital Association, yearly.

Directory of Multihospital Systems (Chicago: American Hospital Association, 1980).

Directory of Investor-Owned Hospitals and Hospital Management Companies (Little Rock, Arkansas: Federation of American Hospitals, 1980).

3 AMBULATORY CARE

Strictly speaking, the term *ambulatory care* refers to care rendered to patients who come to physicians' offices, outpatient departments, and health centers. However, it often includes other non-inpatient components of care such as emergency and home care services. The term is also often used synonymously with *community medicine*. This field is complex and many of its aspects are rapidly changing. The following are brief descriptions of components that are of particular importance or current interest.

FORMS OF PHYSICIAN PRACTICE

Solo Practice. This is an independent practice by a physician usually using his or her own facilities and equipment, but sometimes sharing these with one or more other physicians. There are also usually informal interphysician arrangements for mutual after hours and vacation coverage. A formal arrangement for using common facilities is often termed an *association*. Legally, a solo practitioner is a *sole proprietor*, one owner of an unincorporated business. (A sole proprietorship can also include one or more physicians employed by the physician owner.) Solo practice is a steadily declining but still important form of practice.

Partnership. This is a legal agreement between two or more physicians to share income and assets in an unincorporated business, with each partner legally the agent of the other. (Many group practices are in fact partnerships.) Physicians joining an established practice may work for a time under a salary or other arrangements before being admitted to the partnership. There may be senior and junior partners.

Group Practice. There is no one generally accepted definition of group practice, but a widely accepted common denominator is a voluntary association of three or more physicians in medical practice who use common facilities and share income in a designated way. It is not a legally defined entity.

The American Medical Association (AMA) defines a group practice as "the application of medical services by three or more physicians formally organized to provide medical care, consultation, diagnosis and/or treatment through the joint use of equipment and personnel, and with the income from medical practice distributed in accordance with methods previously determined by members of the group." Groups so defined consist of three categories:

1. Single specialty groups
2. General/family practice groups
3. Multispecialty groups (providing services in at least two specialties)

The first group practice, a multispecialty group, was the well-known Mayo Clinic, which developed in Rochester, Minnesota in the decade after 1900.[1] Group practices began to develop in significant numbers in the 1920s, particularly in the West and Midwest, but their growth was relatively slow. There has been a more rapid increase beginning after World War II, especially in single specialty groups.

The 1975 AMA survey of medical groups[2] denoted 8,483 group practices involving about 67,000 physicians. Slightly more than half

1. The Mayo Clinic group was well-established by 1914 and grew rapidly thereafter. It developed out of the very successful partnership of William Mayo and his sons William and Charles — a partnership established in 1887 as a primarily surgical practice.

2. Louis J. Goodman, Edward H. Bennett, and Richard J. Odem, *Group Medical Practice in the United States, 1975* (Center for Health Services Research and Development, American Medical Association, 1976).

(54.2 percent) were single specialty groups of which the specialties most commonly represented were internists, radiologists, and orthopedic surgeons. In 1980 there were 1,762 group practices involving 88,290 physicians. Of these groups 57.2 percent were single specialty groups.[3]

Some of the larger group practices are associated with prepayment plans; among these are the Permanente groups in California (Kaiser Foundation Health Plan) and the HIP (Health Insurance Plan of Greater New York). Such "prepaid group practices" are now usually discussed under the rubric *health maintenance organizations*, or HMOs (see page 112).

Physicians practice in groups in many organized settings under a variety of salary and other arrangements. These include health centers, outpatient departments, health maintenance organizations, and industrial health departments. Whether such physicians are in formal "group practice" is often a matter of definition and semantics.

Associations:

American Group Practice Association[4]
Medical Group Management Association[5]
Group Health Association of America
   (prepaid group practice health plans)

Professional Corporation.   This is a legal entity that is distinct from its members. There is limited liability for corporate debts, but physician members remain liable for their own negligent acts. Professional corporations are organized under state professional corporation or professional association acts and are now permitted in all states.[6] A series of court decisions led the Internal Revenue Service in 1969 to recognize such corporations for tax purposes. This, together with the abolition by many states of prohibitions against such corporate practice, has resulted in a significant increase in their number, largely because of tax-related financial advantages. In the 1975 AMA survey, 61 percent of groups were so organized, compared with 15.7 percent

3. Preliminary data for the 1980 survey are reviewed in "The Changing Structure of Group Medical Practice in the United States 1969–1980," Larry J. Freshnock and Lynn E. Jensen, *Journal of the American Medical Association* 21 (June 5, 1981): 2173–2176.

4. Formerly American Association of Medical Clinics.

5. Formerly National Association of Clinic Managers.

6. They are denoted by initials such as P.C., P.A., and Inc. Legally the physicians are considered employees of the corporation.

in 1969. In the 1980 survey 70.6 percent were incorporated. Solo practitioners as well as groups of physicians may be incorporated.

"Private Practice." This is generally understood to mean independent practice by physicians (solo, partnership, group) in which patients pay fees for care rendered ("fee for service"). Mutual free choice of physician and patient is also implied. Physicians in group practice contracting with prepaid plans may also, variably, be considered private practitioners.

AMBULATORY CARE CENTERS, PROGRAMS, AND AGENCIES

Outpatient Departments. These are hospital departments where persons not requiring hospitalization may receive care. In the past often termed "dispensary,"[7] it is now apt to be called an "ambulatory care service." The outpatient department is usually distinguished from the emergency room, although persons with nonurgent problems are often seen in the latter area, especially during hours when the outpatient unit is not open. It is commonly referred to as the *clinic*, as are its component units (i.e., medical clinic, surgical clinic). The term "clinic" is also often used for large group practices, such as the Mayo Clinic.

The population served is generally a low-income one, although middle-income persons may be served, especially at university teaching hospitals, and special consultation mechanisms may be available for referring physicians. In the past, patients have usually been seen by house staff (interns and residents) or unpaid attending physicians (voluntary staff), but these arrangements have been changing. Private patients may be seen by physicians who have offices at the hospital under rental or other arrangements. This is usually distinguished from the general outpatient department by a term such as "private ambulatory service."

Many outpatient departments are being reorganized along group practice models, and their administrative and financial relationships

7. Dispensaries were originally independent charitable entities for the treatment of sick poor. They developed for the most part in parallel with hospitals and were ultimately displaced by hospital outpatient departments.

with the hospitals of which they are a part have been undergoing many changes.[8] In particular, there has been a widespread trend toward the organization of medical practice groups by full-time medical school faculty sponsored by the schools and their teaching hospitals, usually according to specialty departments ("academic group practice"). Financial and other relationships vary. Some such groups have been incorporated as independent or quasi-independent entities.[9]

Health Centers. This term has been used to refer to the locus of a wide variety of health care and related activities, and generally implies services to a specific local area, district, or neighborhood. In the past it has most commonly meant a unit of a city or county health department, housing preventive services such as well-child and prenatal clinics, and venereal disease and tuberculosis control and treatment units. The term is now used more broadly to include many community-based centers such as neighborhood health centers.

Neighborhood Health Centers (Community Health Centers). These are health centers whose purpose is to provide a program of comprehensive health services to a defined (urban) local area, often with related social services, and generally with some degree (often considerable), of involvement and participation of members of the local community. The use of nontraditional personnel such as family health workers,[10] and emphasis on "health care teams" have been characteristic of many of these centers.

8. Many of the financial issues are well reviewed by Richard A. Berman and Thomas W. Maloney in "Are Outpatient Departments Responsible for the Fiscal Crisis Facing Teaching Hospitals?" *Journal of Ambulatory Care Management* (January 1978): 37–53.

9. The Association of American Medical Colleges has surveyed sixty-seven of these practices in *Medical Practice Plans at U.S. Medical Schools: A Review of Current Characteristics and Trends;* (interim Final Report, 1977), See also "Medical Practice Plans"—papers by B. Siegal and P. Mancino in *Journal of Medical Education* 53 (1978): 791–799.

10. The family health worker is a health occupation developed at the Dr. Martin Luther King, Jr. Health Center in New York City. [See Harold B. Wise et al., "The Family Health Worker," *American Journal of Public Health* 58 (1968): 1828.] It is representative of a cadre of newly trained, usually previously unskilled workers, typically recruited from the communities served. They carry out a variety of delegated nursing, health education, social service, and social advocacy functions in health centers and the community. Terminology is diverse and includes community health aides, health guides, neighborhood aides, neighborhood health agents, and "outreach" workers. In the setting of changing priorities and levels of federal funding, the numbers of these workers have been declining.

Many neighborhood health centers were developed in the 1960s, largely with federal funding under legislation such as the Economic Opportunity Act,[11] and Title V of the Social Security Act.[12] Many are sponsored by local health department programs and by community groups. Many, including the original OEO centers are now partially funded by the Public Health Service.

Freestanding centers are independent organizations legally governed by community boards. A "backup" hospital is one that provides specialized services and hospital admissions for these centers. Other centers are legally a part of a hospital or health department and operate under that institution's governing board and license and have advisory community boards. Many of these centers actually function with considerable autonomy; their advisory boards may have certain defined powers in the area of general and personnel policies delegated by agreement with the governing institution. Others function as decentralized outpatient department units or satellite clinics.

Rural Health Centers. Analogous to the urban health centers are the rural health centers developed under federal financing (migrant health, Appalachian development, and the Economic Opportunity Act) by health departments and community groups, sometimes with foundation support. Since they are typically located in poor areas with few physicians they are especially notable for their use of nurse practitioners and physician's assistants linked to physicians in other sites. A recent federal statute[13] provides for Medicare and Medicaid reimbursement of such personnel in certain centers without full-time physicians.

Mental Health Centers (Community Mental Health Centers). These centers emphasize the provision of a wide range of mental health services in the community, usually to a defined geographical "catchment" area, rather than the treatment of hospitalized patients. A community mental health center need not be a single physical entity; it can actually be a network of coordinated services. Teams are also

---

11. Funded the OEO (Office of Economic Opportunity) neighborhood health centers, which were the origins of the recent neighborhood health center movement.

12. Maternity and Infant Care, Children and Youth Projects.

13. Rural Health Clinic Services Act, PL 95–210 (1977).

often emphasized here, as well as short-term and "crisis interven-tion" approaches to treatment.

The centers may be sponsored by state mental health departments or psychiatric departments of hospitals,[14] or they may be indepen-dent nonprofit entities. They may be separate physical facilities or may operate as a part of, or a replacement for, outpatient psychiatric services. They have available inpatient beds, either as an integral part of the center or through an affiliated mental hospital or psychiatric unit of a general hospital.

The term "community mental health center" is often used to refer to centers that have received funding under the Community Men-tal Health Center Act (see Chapter 6) and have met federal require-ments for comprehensive services. Over 750 centers have received such funding. There are, however, other community mental health centers that have not been federally assisted and that offer a spec-trum of community-oriented mental health services. Some antedate the federal legislation reflecting the movement toward community mental health, of which this legislation was one aspect.

Drug Rehabilitation Programs. Programs for rehabilitation of drug abusers include *methadone maintenance programs*, hospital-related programs for heroin addicts based on the long-term use of meth-adone as a heroin substitute, supplemented in varying degrees by other rehabilitative services; and *drug-free* programs. The drug-free programs comprise a diverse group, including programs in mental health units; halfway houses; residential therapeutic communities;[15] and a variety of self-help residential programs (e.g., Synanon), coun-seling centers, and "hot-lines."

"Free Clinics." These are neighborhood clinics that provide medical services in relatively informal settings and styles to, generally, stu-dents, transient youth, and minority groups. Care is given at no or nominal charge by predominantly volunteer staffs. The first such clinic is considered to be the Haight–Ashbury Free Clinic, organized in San Francisco in the summer of 1967 by David Smith. Their num-

---

14. One aspect of the community mental health movement has been the development of psychiatric units in general hospitals.

15. A notable example is *Oddyssey House*, which operates thirteen residential therapeu-tic communities in five states. It is a division of Oddyssey Institute, a nonprofit organization that carries out many activities related to the prevention and treatment of drug abuse.

bers reached a peak of perhaps 400 (estimates vary) in the early 1970s. Some did not survive and many have evolved toward more formally organized health centers with various sources of funding.

Women's Clinics. These are health units developed and operated by women that address a variety of women's health problems. They have grown out of the women's movement coupled with the consumer activism and self-help movements. Many developed from free clinics. Great emphasis is placed on health promotion, group participation, and use of lay health workers. Services include, variably, routine gynecological care, birth control, maternity care, and general health care. The women involved range from declared feminists to middle- and working-class women concerned primarily about securing personal health care in a noninstitutional, relatively deprofessionalized, mutually supportive setting.

Professionals at these clinics are variably involved in educational, consultation, and service capacities. Some clinics participate in "alternative delivery systems" such as birthing centers and home births, including the use of nurse-midwives and in a few instances, lay midwives. The first such clinic is generally considered to be the Feminist Women's Center of Los Angeles, established in 1973.

The *National Women's Health Network* addresses issues related to women's health.

Birth Centers (Birthing Centers, Alternative Birth Centers). These are out-of-hospital centers for prenatal care and delivery of women expected to have normal pregnancies. They have developed as an alternative to both the traditional hospital environment of labor and delivery, and home births, which, though few in number, have been increasing in many states. These centers emphasize a homelike atmosphere, natural childbirth techniques, and family orientation. They are generally staffed by nurse midwives with consultation and assistance as needed from obstetricians.

The first two such centers established (1975), were the Childbearing Center in New York City (sponsored by the Maternity Center Association) and the Southwest Maternity Center in Albuquerque, New Mexico. A parallel and more rapid development has been the establishment in many hospitals of similar centers, often with the participation of nurse-midwives.

Family Planning Clinics. These are clinics that provide a spectrum of birth control services. Most notable are the 700 clinics of the Planned Parenthood Federation (one of the oldest and largest of the voluntary agencies in the health field).

Abortion Clinics. These have rapidly developed in the last decade since the legalization of abortion, first by many states and then by the Supreme Court in 1973. Sponsorship is quite varied and includes family-planning agencies, community groups, women's clinics, and proprietary organizations.

Short-Stay Surgical Centers ("Surgicenters"). These are independent proprietary facilities for surgical procedures that do not require overnight hospitalization. The principal rationale for the centers is the reduction in costs compared with hospitalization. The first established and best known is the Surgicenter in Phoenix, established in 1970 by two anesthesiologists, John Ford and Wallace Reid. Some are specialized for certain procedures such as plastic surgery. Their numbers have been gradually increasing although approval by Blue Cross plans and regulatory agencies has varied considerably from state to state. A parallel and more rapid development has been an increase in hospital-based outpatient surgery units.

Renal Dialysis Centers. These are centers for the treatment of patients with chronic kidney disease who require periodic use of the "artificial kidney." Many are free standing, mostly physician-owned or developed proprietary organizations.[16] Dialysis units have also been established in many hospitals. The growth of these centers was spurred greatly by the inclusion of persons needing such treatment in the Medicare program (1972 amendments). Many units, especially those based in hospitals also operate home dialysis programs.

Rehabilitation Centers. These are centers that provide a wide spectrum of services for the physical and vocational rehabilitation of handicapped persons. Many include *sheltered workshops.* They may be freestanding or a part of inpatient rehabilitation centers.

16. A notable example is National Medical Care, Inc., which operates over 130 dialysis centers throughout the country.

Visiting Nurse Associations (Visiting Nurse Services). These are voluntary agencies that provide nursing and other services in the home, including health supervision, education, and counseling; bedside care; and the carrying out of physicians' treatment orders. They are staffed by public health nurses and often by other personnel such as nurse practitioners, physiotherapists, speech therapists, and home health aides. The latter are specially trained to provide services such as bedside and personal care, assistance with ambulation and exercises, and meal preparation.[17]

These agencies had their origin in the visiting or "district" nursing provided to sick poor in their homes by voluntary agencies, such as the New York City Mission, in the 1870s. The first visiting nurse associations were established in Buffalo, Boston, and Philadelphia in 1886 and 1887.

Health Department Nursing Units. In many communities public health nurses from local health departments provide nursing services in the home. Particularly in areas without visiting nurse associations, they provide similar services, although traditionally they have carried out health department functions in the area of maternal and child health, and communicable disease control. As with visiting nurse associations, they may employ other types of personnel.

Combined Agencies. These are nursing agencies jointly staffed by nurses from both voluntary (i.e., visiting nurse associations) and "official" agencies (i.e., city or county health departments).

Home Care Programs. These are organized programs, hospital or community-based, for the provision of a spectrum of health-related services, equipment, and supplies to patients in their homes, generally patients with chronic illness. Community-based programs usually supplement the services of private practitioners; hospital-based programs may provide physician services. The earliest home care program, and still among the best known, was established in 1947 at Montefiore Hospital in New York City.

---

17. Homemakers who are generally employed by social welfare agencies perform many similar functions, but are apt to assume more responsibility for management of the home, often in the setting of family crises, such as the hospitalization of a mother.

Home Health Agencies. This is a term defined in federal legislation (see p. 313) referring to an agency authorized to receive payment under the federal Medicare program for services provided in the home. Organizations certified as home health agencies include visiting nurse associations, units of local health departments, and home care programs.

A number of proprietary agencies have been established to provide the home services of personnel such as home health aides and practical nurses. Some are subsidiary chains of companies such as the Upjohn Corporation. Until recently, they were not eligible to participate in Medicare unless they were state licensed. Under 1980 federal legislation they are now eligible if they meet the conditions for participation for home health agencies.

Hospices. This is a general term for programs of supportive and palliative services for patients who are terminally ill, usually with cancer. This may be a specialized form of home care, with emphasis on support and supplementation of family efforts, including the use of volunteers and visiting nurses, social workers, clergy, and others. The first hospice in the United States was established in 1974, in New Haven, Connecticut, through the efforts of Sylvia Lack. This was initially a home hospice,[18] using techniques and approaches for the dying patient developed by Cicely Saunders and her associates at the freestanding St. Christopher Hospice in London. St. Christopher's, established in 1967, was designed specifically to create a homelike environment. Now, in addition to home hospice programs, freestanding and hospital-based units are also being rapidly developed.

Emergency Services. Emergency services are for the most part provided by organized departments of hospitals with immediate, prehospital care provided by a variety of ambulance and rescue services operated by police and fire departments, volunteers, and commercial ambulance companies. In many areas these services are being coordinated into regional *emergency medical systems* with federal and state funding and regulation.[19] These systems often include the categoriza-

18. The hospice now includes a specially designed freestanding inpatient unit in Branden, Connecticut, near New Haven.

19. The development of these systems has been spurred by federal grants under the Emergency Medical Services Systems Act and by requirements under the National Highway Safety Act.

tion of emergency rooms according to their capabilities (determined by personnel and services available) and in some instances the designation of specific hospitals and their emergency rooms as specialized centers, such as trauma centers and burn centers.

Special emphasis has been on prehospital services including the improvement of communications and equipment and the training of ambulance personnel. Large numbers of *emergency medical technicians* (EMTs) have been trained. Many *paramedics* (advanced EMTs, EMT IIs) have also been trained; they staff an increasing number of highly-equipped *mobile intensive care units* (MICUs).

Emergency Centers (Emergicenters). A recent development has been the establishment in many areas of freestanding emergency clinics for the immediate "walk-in" treatment of non-life-threatening acute illnesses. These are in many ways analogous to the "surgicenters" in that they offer an alternative to the hospital, in this case the hospital emergency room.

SPECIAL AMBULATORY CARE PERSONNEL

Public Health Nurse (Community Health Nurse)[20]

A public health nurse generally works in the community and is concerned with the health of groups and persons in their usual environment such as home, school, or work. These nurses are most often based in health departments, schools, or voluntary agencies such as visiting nurse associations. They traditionally function relatively independently and tend to be oriented especially toward the community, the family, and the promotion of health and normal development.

Training includes experience in a community agency, either during a baccalaureate nursing program (as field experience) or after graduation from nursing school. Advanced training formerly obtained by special courses granting a certificate is now obtained via master's degree programs.

---

20. For a good discussion of public health nursing, see John J. Hanlon and George E. Pickett, "Community Nursing Services," in *Public Health Administration and Practice*, 7th ed. (St. Louis: The C. V. Mosby Company, 1979).

Nurse Practitioner

This is a registered nurse who has received additional training in clinical skills, including assessment and management of certain illnesses.

Pediatric Nurse Practitioner (Pediatric Nurse Associate). A pediatric nurse practitioner is a registered nurse who has been trained, in a program of four months' (or more) duration, to assume an expanded role in the care of children. This includes comprehensive well-child care, and the appraisal and management of certain conditions of the acute or chronically ill child. The first formal training program was developed in 1967 by Henry K. Silver and Loretta C. Ford at the Schools of Medicine and Nursing of the University of Colorado. Many programs of varying lengths were then quickly established, often with the assistance of federal funding. The general trend recently has been toward master's degree programs.

Other Practitioners. More recently, training programs have been developed for "adult (medical) nurse practitioners," "family nurse practitioners," and other specialties. These also include master's degree programs.

Legal Recognition. The activities of nurse practitioners are generally considered as aspects of nursing practice, and specific new licensing legislation has not been pursued. However, the general trend toward expanded nursing roles has led many states in the past few years to amend their nursing practice acts to broaden the definition of nursing practice; some amendments have included language directed to nurse practitioners.

Certification. The American Nursing Association certifies nurse practitioners. Pediatric nurse practitioners may also be certified by the National Board of Pediatric Nurse Practitioners and Assistants, in cooperation with the American Academy of Pediatrics.

Physician Extenders

This term refers to types of health personnel trained to extend the capabilities of physicians, especially in situations of physician shortage. This may be by direct assistance or by substitution in the performance of certain tasks and services.

Physician's Assistant (PA).   A physician's assistant is trained to perform a variety of routine and delegated patient services under the supervision or direction of a physician. The first formal training program was established at Duke University in 1966 by Eugene A. Stead. The Duke program comprises nine months' formal instruction and fifteen months in clinical rotations, a format that has been characteristic of many subsequent programs.

Most physician's assistants are generalist-trained; the American Medical Association, which participates in program accreditation, calls them *assistants to the primary care physician.* Other types of physician's assistants being developed include *surgeon's assistants, orthopedic physician's assistants,* and *urological physician's assistants.*

Legal Recognition.   Most states now recognize physician's assistants in amendments to medical practice acts. Such statutes make explicit the authority of the physician to delegate functions, or provide for specific regulation by bodies such as boards of medical examiners or registration. In some instances the specific physician supervising the physician's assistant must be named, and often the number that may be supervised by one physician is restricted.

Certification.   Physician's assistants are certified by the *National Commission on Certification of Physician's Assistants.*

MEDEX.[21]   MEDEX programs are physician's assistant programs that were developed specifically for former medical corpsmen with independent duty experience. Their purpose was to train extensions for physicians, especially for general practitioners in rural areas. (Most MEDEX have been trained to work with specific physicians.) The first such program was begun in 1969 by Richard A. Smith at the University of Washington, in cooperation with the Washington State Medical Association. The programs generally consist of three months of university training and twelve months of preceptorship.

---

21. From the French, *médecin extension.*

Child Health Associate. This program was begun in 1969 at the University of Colorado to train child care professionals capable of handling a variety of non-life-threatening pediatric problems. This is a five-year program leading to a bachelor of science degree and includes two years of undergraduate work, two years at the medical center, and one year of internship.

Nurse Practitioner. Nurse practitioners (see above) are sometimes considered in the physician extender category.

SPECIAL TERMS

Comprehensive Care. This is a system that provides a wide variety of health care services, with the implication that these will be coordinated under the overall direction of a responsible physician or "team" of professionals, with appropriate attention to preventive and rehabilitative services and socioeconomic factors.

Primary Care. This is a not yet well-defined term that has gained wide currency since the term *primary physician* was proposed in the report of the Citizens' Commission on Graduate Education in 1966.[22] Its meaning varies from that of "first contact" care (often with the implication of care simple to render, or of evaluation/referral) to that of broad, continuing responsibility for care of individuals or families. In many contexts it has replaced the older term "comprehensive care." It often implies the treatment of common illnesses. It may also be used as the opposite of specialty or subspecialty care. It is probably most often used to denote the care usually rendered by family practitioners, internists, or pediatricians.[23]

By extension, the term *tertiary care* has come into wide use. It is rarely defined but generally implies highly specialized, highly technological care rendered in large teaching hospitals, especially university hospitals. *Secondary care*, a term used less often, variably means care

22. *The Graduate Education of Physicians*, popularly known as the "Millis Report" after the commission chairman, John S. Millis. The term was used to denote a physician who would be specially trained to provide comprehensive, continuing health care. It is now often used as a generic term to refer to general or family practitioners, internists, and pediatricians.

23. A staff paper for the National Institute of Medicine's Committee on Primary Care Manpower analyzed thirty-eight definitions of primary care.

by specialists or subspecialists, care intermediate between routine primary care and very sophisticated tertiary care, or care in other than tertiary care hospitals. Some speak of *primary care hospitals*, but there are few, if any, active candidates for this designation.

Triage.[24]   This term is now commonly used to describe the sorting out or screening of patients seeking care, to determine which service is initially required, and with what priority. A patient coming to a facility for care may be seen in a "triage," "screening," or "walk-in" clinic. Here it will be determined, possibly by a "triage nurse" or nurse practitioner, for example, whether the patient has a medical or surgical problem or requires some nonphysician service, such as social service consultation. Such rapid assessment units may merely refer patients to the most appropriate treatment service, but frequently they will also give treatment. They are a feature of organizationally complex systems such as emergency and outpatient departments and health maintenance organizations.

Deinstitutionalization.   This is the discharge of patients from state institutions for the mentally ill and mentally retarded to care in the community by community mental health centers, halfway houses, and other resources. This policy has become a very controversial one in many communities, especially large cities where insufficient preparations have been made and too few resources established to handle the large numbers of formerly institutionalized persons. Many are now housed in nursing homes, residential hotels, and proprietary homes for adults.

The trend toward deinstitutionalization had its origins in the concepts of community psychiatry which emerged in the 1950s, the development of antipsychotic drugs, also in the 1950s, and the development of federally supported community mental health centers in the 1960s. Also contributing to the trend, especially in certain states, has been the economic incentive of cost transfer from the states (mental hospitals) to partially or fully federally funded programs such as Medicaid and SSI (Supplemental Security Income).

---

24. From the French, "selecting, sifting," originally applied medically to the sorting of battle casualties.

Appointment System. This is the arrangement whereby a patient is given a definite time and date for a visit. *Block appointments* are those given for the same time to several patients. *Staggered appointments* are those given to each patient for a specific separate time during a session. These are also referred to as "wave" and "stream" systems. "Walk-in" refers to a patient who comes in for care without an appointment.

Screening, Multiphasic Screening. This is frequently an adjunct of ambulatory care programs; a system whereby a variety of routine tests are performed for the purpose of early disease detection.

Automated Multiphasic Health Testing (AMHT). This is a highly organized system of health testing that includes the use of automated equipment and data processing techniques. These are largely a feature of some health maintenance organizations (HMOs) and proprietary screening centers that offer these services to physicians for their patients.

VOLUME OF PHYSICIAN VISITS

Despite the increase in alternative ambulatory care programs such as community health centers, the great majority of physician visits take place in physician's offices and hospital outpatient departments. According to the 1975 Health Interview Survey, there were nearly one billion annual visits to physicians (exclusive of inpatients), an average of about five per person. Of these 77.6 percent were in physicians' offices, 14.8 percent were in hospital clinics or emergency rooms, and .9 percent were at home.[25]

25. U.S. Department of Health, Education and Welfare, "Physican Visits – Volume and Interval since Last Visit, United States, 1975," *Vital and Health Statistics*, Series 10, no. 128, data from the National Health Survey, National Center for Health Statistics, 1979.

SELECTED READINGS

"Private Medical Group Practice," in *Ambulatory Health Services in America: Past, Present, and Future*, Milton I. Roemer (Gaithersburg, Maryland: Aspen Systems Corporation, 1981).

Health and the War on Poverty: A Ten-Year Appraisal, Karen Davis and Kathy Schoen (Washington, D.C.: The Brookings Institution, 1978).

"Outreach in Urban Clinics," Frederick P. Rivera, *Journal of Community Health* 6 (1980): 43.

"Mental Health Services," Lorrin M. Koran. In *Health Care Delivery in the United States*, 2nd. ed., Steven Jonas and contributors (New York: Springer Publishing Company, 1981).

"The Pediatric Nurse Practitioner Program: Expanding the Role of the Nurse to Provide Increased Health Care for Children," Henry K. Silver, Loretta C. Ford, and Lewis R. Day, *Journal of the American Medical Association*, 204 (1968): 298.

"The Law and the Expanded Nursing Role," Bonnie Bullough, *Journal of the American Public Health Association*, 66 (1976): 249.

"Conserving Costly Talents—Providing Physicians New Assistants," Eugene A. Stead, *Journal of the American Medical Association*, 198 (1966): 1108.

"MEDEX," Richard A. Smith, *Journal of the American Medical Association*, 211 (1970): 1843.

4 HEALTH MANPOWER

The health care "industry" is labor intensive—requiring large numbers of personnel. As it continues to expand and to make increasing use of technology it requires not only greater numbers of manpower but more specialized skills. There are now over 200 occupations in the health field, including many professions, and new ones are constantly appearing. Table 4–1 lists some of these occupations and Table 4–2 estimates the total number of personnel within selected health care occupations. The total number of people employed in health services rose from 4.2 million in 1970 to 6.8 million in 1979 (see Table 4–3).

The word "professional" has no consistent or agreed upon meaning. Most occupational groups in the health field aspire to being considered professions. There are a number of components to the definition of a profession.[1]

- Formal education and examination are required for membership in the profession.

1. See Ernest Greenwood, "Attributes of a Profession," in S. Noscow and W. Form, eds., *Man, Work, and Society* (New York: Basic Books, 1962) and Eliot Freidson, *Profession of Medicine* (New York: Dodd Mead & Co., 1970).

61

- Certification or licensure is required for membership, reflecting community sanction or approval.
- There are regional or national associations.
- There is a code of ethics.
- There is a body of systematic scientific knowledge and technical skill required.
- The members function with a degree of autonomy and authority, under the assumption that they alone have the expertise to make decisions in their area of competence.

Medicine (in the sense of physician practice) is often considered the occupation that most closely approaches the prototype of a profession.

In actuality there is no clear-cut distinction between professions and nonprofessions or between professionals and nonprofessionals; rather, there is a continuum as occupations become professionalized.[2] The term "semiprofession" has been used, but not widely accepted, for occupations that do not have all the characteristics of a profession.[3]

A number of other somewhat ill-defined terms are used in relation to health manpower, not all of which are accepted by those being referred to. *Paraprofessional* or *ancillary* personnel refer to those who work alongside a professional and *subprofessional* refers to occupations that are subordinate to other professions. *Allied health personnel* are those who work with physicians; this category usually includes all hospital personnel, but excludes, for example, independent practitioners such as dentists, podiatrists, pharmacists, optometrists, and chiropractors.

2. The American Heritage Dictionary defines "profession" as "an occupation or vocation requiring training in the liberal arts or the sciences and advanced study in a specialized field" and a professional as "one who has an assured competence in a particular field or occupation."

3. Amitai Etzioni, ed., *The Semi-Professions and Their Organization* (Glencoe, Ill.: The Free Press, 1961).

The terms *technologist, therapist, technician, assistant,* and *aide* are accepted but are now used in no systematic way. The following definitions have been suggested: [4]

Technologist Therapist	Requires education at, or above, the baccalaureate level
Technician Assistant	Requires education at, or beyond, the two-year college level (the associate degree level)
Aide	Requires less than two years beyond high school or on-the-job training

Needless to say, there is not enough room to address all the health occupations. A representative number have been selected for description. We hope our readers will understand that even though this chapter does not describe groups such as psychiatric art therapists and marine physician's assistants (serving U.S. Merchant Marine sailors at sea), they have important roles and responsibilities. In the sections that follow there will be more space devoted to physicians and nurses because these health occupations are most frequently referred to, and their education is often used as a standard to compare with that of other professional groups.

REGULATION

Regulation is here being used in the broad sense of both governmental and voluntary nongovernmental activities.

Certification, Registration, and Licensure [5]

Certification is the process by which a nongovernmental agency or association grants recognition to an individual who has certain predetermined qualifications specified by that agency or association. A

---

4. *Health Resources Statistics, 1972*, U.S. Department of Health, Education, and Welfare, Health Services and Mental Health Administration (Rockville, Md.: National Center for Health Statistics, February 1972).

5. These definitions are based on those in *Health Resources Statistics, 1976–77*, U.S. Department of Health, Education and Welfare; Health Services and Mental Health Administration (Rockville, Md.: National Center for Health Statistics, 1977). For additional definitions and comments on certification, registration, licensure, and accreditation, see Chapter 9.

diplomate is one certified by an agency recognized as professionally competent to grant such certification.

Registration is the process by which qualified individuals are listed on an official roster maintained by a governmental or nongovernmental agency. Registration in some cases allows the individual to use a designation after his or her name. For example, a cytotechnologist registered by the Board of Registry of the American Society of Clinical Pathologists may use the designation CT (ASCP).

Licensure is the process by which an agency of government grants permission to persons meeting predetermined qualifications to engage in a given occupation and/or use a particular title. Legislation usually establishes educational experience and personal qualifications, requires successful completion of an examination, and provides issuance of a license as a prior condition for entrance into the occupation.

As of 1977, thirty-five health professions were licensed in one or more states.[6] Licensed in all states are chiropractors, dental hygienists, dentists, environmental health engineers, optometrists, pharmacists, physical therapists, medical and osteopathic physicians, nursing home administrators, podiatrists, practical nurses, psychologists, registered nurses, and veterinarians. Some states license clinical laboratory directors (nineteen), dental laboratory technicians (one), medical technologists (ten), midwives (twenty-three), nurse midwives (seven), ophthalmic laboratory technicians (two), opticians (seventeen), physical therapy assistants (fourteen), physician's assistants (one), psychiatric aides (three), psychologists (forty-seven), radiologic technologists (three), respiratory therapists (one), sanitarians (thirty-five), sanitarian technicians (one), social workers (eleven), and speech pathologists and audiologists (fourteen).

Approval and Accreditation of Educational Programs

The states approve many educational programs leading to licensed professions. This is usually done by the state's department of education on boards of registration. There is usually *reciprocity* between states which allows graduates from one state to be eligible for licensure in another state.

---

6. *Ibid.*

Accreditation is a means of nongovernmental evaluation and recognition of educational institutions. It can be concerned with an institution as a whole or a specialized part of an institution. The Secretary of Education publishes a list of recognized accrediting agencies for the purpose of determining institutional eligibility for federal programs of assistance. Otherwise, the federal government does not exercise control over private educational institutions. State control varies substantially and, in general, private institutions of higher education function with considerable autonomy.

The Council on Postsecondary Accreditation is a private, independent agency whose members include colleges and universities that grants recognition to qualified, voluntary accrediting agencies. In the health field, the American Medical Association (AMA), plays a major role in accrediting educational programs. Its representatives participate in the accreditation of medical schools and, with over forty other collaborating organizations, its Committee on Allied Health Education and Accreditation (CAHEA) accredits educational programs for twenty-four allied health occupations. Table 4-4 lists those agencies and organizations that accredit educational programs for selected occupations.

PHYSICIANS

Physician (MD) Education

The educational requirements for the training of physicians was largely cast in its present mold as a result of the "Flexner Report"[7] in 1910, in which Abraham Flexner criticized many of the medical schools of his day. As a result the American Medical Association undertook the accreditation of medical schools, classifying them as "A," "B," or "C," depending on their performance. Since 1938 only "A" rated medical schools have existed.

The most common path to becoming a physician is as follows: four years of college including a number of *premedical* courses including biology, chemistry, organic chemistry, and physics; taking the required Medical College Admissions Test (MCAT), which is used

---

7. Abraham Flexner, *Medical Education in the United States and Canada*, A Report to the Carnegie Foundation for the Advancement of Teaching (New York: The Carnegie Foundation, 1910).

to help evaluate the applicant's potential; four years of medical school, which are usually divided into two preclinical or basic science years and two clinical years, the latter largely in affiliated teaching hospitals; and usually several years of *residency training* in a teaching hospital. The MD degree is awarded at the completion of medical school.

Education in medical school is referred to as *undergraduate medical education*, and the residency years are *graduate medical education* (GME). Short courses taken throughout later life are called *continuing medical education* (CME).

Medical School (Undergraduate Medical Education). There are 126 medical schools, two of which provide only the first two years of basic medical sciences, after which students may transfer with advanced standing to a four-year school. Medical schools are accredited by the Liaison Committee on Medical Education (LCME), which is composed of representatives of the AMA (six), the Association of American Medical Colleges (six), the Association of Canadian Medical Colleges (two), the public (two), and the federal government (one). With a few hospital-based exceptions, medical schools are either state or privately owned, and part of a university. Some own and operate their own teaching hospitals, others have contractual affiliation agreements with independent hospitals, and others have both. The *Association of American Medical Colleges* (AAMC) is the major national representative association of medical schools.

In recent years some schools have developed variations from the standard medical school curriculum. For example, there are a number of concentrated three-year programs (fewer in number however than in 1973) and several six-year programs that combine college and medical school. There is a shortened program for students with doctoral degrees (University of Miami) and some medical schools have tracks that lead to the MD and PhD or other graduate degrees concurrently.

Because of the limited number of places in U.S. medical schools, over 10,000 Americans are studying abroad. Most of these are now enrolled in ten schools in Mexico (notably the University of Guadalajara) and the Caribbean. Many of these are newly established and accept mostly, and in some cases exclusively, U.S. citizens. Americans also continue to enroll in schools in Italy, Spain, France, and elsewhere. Some students succeed after two years in transferring with advanced standing to U.S. schools.

Graduate Medical Education. Residency (graduate medical education) can vary from three to seven years depending on the specialty chosen. Until recently, the first year of graduate training was called the *internship* and a distinction was made between internship and residency programs. These have now been combined as unified residencies. These training years are also called *postgraduate years* as in "first postgraduate year" (PGY-1). After the completion of the first residency year the physician is eligible to apply for state licensure. There are about 5,000 residency programs in 1,700 hospitals. Initial selection into a residency program is made through the National Resident Matching Program (NRMP), which uses a computerized program to match applicant and hospital preferences. Figure 4-1 shows the required residency training for the twenty-three specialties. Some specialty training starts in the first year, such as pediatrics and general surgery. Other specialties start after a general first year in internal medicine or surgery, such as neurology and orthopedic surgery.

Residency programs are accredited by the Accreditation Council on Graduate Medical Education (ACGME), which is composed of representatives of the AMA (four), AAMC (four), American Hospital Association (two), American Board of Medical Specialties (four), Council of Medical Specialty Societies (two), and a representative of the federal government, the public, and residents. Additional training is sometimes obtained by means of fellowships of one or more years. These are not accredited and therefore vary greatly in their content.

Specialization. After specialty training a physician may become a *board certified specialist*. Legally any physician may specialize without certification. A physician who has completed the required residency training but not passed the specialty board examination is called *board qualified*. When the exam is passed and other qualifications are met the physician is *board certified*, or a *diplomate* of that board. Many specialists then go on to become members or fellows of the *college* associated with their specialty. For example, a board certified surgeon may become a fellow of the American Col-

Figure 4-1. Progression and Duration of Residency Training by Medical Specialty.

The educational sequence toward specialty board certification commonly followed by U.S. graduates during residency training is shown. The "general year" shown for the support specialties may be either a flexible program (one sponsored by two or more residency programs) or a year in a broad specialty such as internal medicine or surgery. Over half of the graduates who enter psychiatry, anesthesiology, and pathology enter their programs directly from medical school.

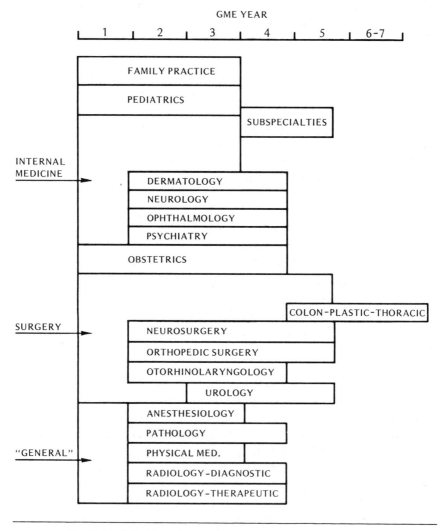

Source: The National Resident Matching Program, Evanston, Illinois.

lege of Surgery, which entitles the surgeon to add these initials after his or her name (for example, Ann Jones, MD, F.A.C.S.).

There are twenty-three American Specialty Boards. They are recognized and approved by the American Board of Medical Specialists in conjunction with the AMA Council on Medical Education. The following are the twenty-three American Medical Specialty Boards in alphabetical order:

1. Allergy and Immunology (formed in 1971), a conjoint board of the American Boards of Internal Medicine and Pediatrics.

2. Anesthesiology (1938).

3. Colon and Rectal Surgery (1935); sometimes this specialty is called Proctology.

4. Dermatology (1932); this can include special certification in dermatopathology.

5. Emergency Medicine (1979), a conjoint board of Surgery, Internal Medicine, Family Practice, Psychology, Obstetrics, Pediatrics, and Otolaryngology plus three emergency medicine groups.

6. Family Practice (1969).

7. Internal Medicine (1936); special certifications include cardiovascular disease, endocrinology, gastroenterology, hematology, infectious disease, medical oncology, nephrology, pulmonary disease, and rheumatology.

8. Neurological Surgery (1940), also called Neurosurgery.

9. Nuclear Medicine (1971), a conjoint board of Internal Medicine, Pathology, Radiology, and The Society for Nuclear Medicine. It provides special certification in radioisotopic pathology and nuclear radiology.

10. Obstetrics and Gynecology (1930); special certification is provided in gynecological oncology, maternal and fetal medicine, and reproductive endocrinology.

11. Ophthalmology (1917); the first specialty board.

12. Orthopedic surgery (1934).

13. Otolaryngology (1924); this specialty is also called ear, nose, and throat (ENT).

14. Pathology (1936); certification is provided in anatomic, clinical, chemical, forensic, and radioisotopic pathology, and blood banking, dermatopathology, hematology, medical microbiology, and neuropathology.

15. Pediatrics (1933); special certification is available in pediatric cardiology, endocrinology, hematology–oncology, nephrology, and neonatal–perinatal medicine.

16. Physical Medicine and Rehabilitation (1947); these specialists are also known as physiatrists.

17. Plastic Surgery (1939).

18. Preventive Medicine (1948); certification is provided in aerospace medicine, general preventive medicine, occupational medicine, and public health.

19. Psychiatry and Neurology (1934); special certification is provided in child psychiatry.

20. Radiology (1934); certification is provided in diagnostic, therapeutic, and nuclear radiology.

21. Surgery (1937); this specialty also is known as General Surgery. Special certification is provided in pediatric surgery.

22. Thoracic Surgery (1948).

23. Urology (1935).

The number of physicians by primary specialty is shown in Table 4–5.

Foreign Medical Graduates (FMGs). In the past, all graduates of foreign medical schools who met the requirements for licensure in the school's country, and who passed the examination given by the Educational Commission for Foreign Medical Graduates (ECFMG)[8] received a certificate permitting them to participate in a U.S. residency program. In 1976, the requirements for entrance to the United States by alien physicians were made more stringent by the Congress. In this setting, foreign medical graduates must now take the Visa Qualifying Examination to qualify for either temporary exchange (J visa)

---

8. The commission is sponsored by the American Hospital Association, the American Medical Association, the Association of American Medical Colleges, the Association for Hospital and Medical Education, and the Federation of State Medical Boards.

or permanent immigrant status. American graduates of foreign medical schools continue to take the ECFMG examinations.

Physician Licensure

Medical licensure is on a state-by-state basis. If a physician is licensed in one state, he or she is not allowed to practice medicine in another state without obtaining its license. (Special temporary state licenses are granted to resident physicians working in hospitals.)

In all states the requirements, which are set forth in Medical Practice Acts, include passing an examination. Traditionally, these have been developed and administered by state boards. In many states, certification by the National Board of Medical Examiners is accepted in lieu of state examinations. Parts I and II of the National Board Examination are taken at the end of the second and fourth years of medical school. Part III is taken during the first residency year. In recent years, there has been wide acceptance by the states of the Federation Licensing Examination (FLEX),[9] developed by the Federation of State Medical Boards. Many states recognize, in lieu of examination, licenses granted by certain other states (reciprocity).

Osteopathic Physicians

Physicians (MDs) and osteopathic physicians (DOs) are often grouped together because their education and mode of practice are similar. Until recently, osteopathy and medicine have constituted separate professions with separate education and hospitals. Recently there has been more interchange between the two.

Osteopathy originated as a reform movement in American medicine, originally propounded in 1874 by Dr. Andrew Taylor Still. It was a system of medical practice that held that musculo-skeletal dysfunctions, especially of the spine, disrupted the body's resistance to disease. It considered medication to be overemphasized by regular physicians. The system has evolved so that osteopathic practitioners now use the diagnostic and therapeutic measures of ordinary medi-

---

9. John P. Hubbard, "Evaluation, Certification and Licensure in Medicine," *Journal of the American Medical Association* 225, 4 (July 23, 1973): 401.

cine in addition to manipulative procedures while maintaining a relatively holistic approach to the patient.

Today there are fifteen colleges of osteopathy accredited by the American Osteopathic Association, whose graduates receive the degree of Doctor of Osteopathy (DO). The content of osteopathic education is the same as that of MD medical schools except that osteopaths have additional class hours devoted to osteopathic manipulation. One year of internship after the DO degree is customary, and beyond that there is further training leading to membership in one of twelve osteopathic specialty boards. While most MDs specialize, most DOs do not. Licensure is required for practice. All states grant osteopathic physicians the same practice privileges as medical physicians. The last state law restricting osteopathic use of drugs and surgery was changed in 1973 (Mississippi).

In 1980 there were 17,700 professionally active osteopathic physicians, up from 10,900 in 1950. Most osteopaths practice in a few states, including Michigan, Missouri, Ohio, Pennsylvania, and Texas. In 1962 the MD and DO professions in California essentially merged and 2,400 osteopathic physicians accepted MD titles from the MD licensing board; a (referendum) law prohibited further licensure of DOs in the state. This law was subsequently declared unconstitutional and the number of osteopathic physicians in California is again increasing.

The word "medicine" is used in three ways. One is to refer to all activities of physicians (as in "the practice of medicine"). The second refers to the specialty of internal medicine, which deals with nonsurgical, nonobstetrical conditions of adults. The third distinguishes medicine from osteopathy. Sometimes osteopathic physicians refer to MDs as *allopathic* physicians.[10]

NURSES

The following is a brief description of nursing, particularly nursing education, which is designed to provide a basic background for the many current issues and changes in the field and its relation to other health professions.

---

10. On the other hand, Dorland's Medical Dictionary (23rd edition) says that allopathy is "an erroneous designation for the regular system of medicine and surgery."

Registered Nurses (RNs)

The term *registered nurse* is generally used in the United States to refer to professionally licensed nurses. In the past the term *graduate nurse* has also been used.

Education. There are three basic types of educational programs that prepare registered nurses: diploma, baccalaureate, and associate degree. In 1978–79 they graduated 77,932 nurses. Nursing education programs are approved by state agencies, usually boards of nursing. In addition, a voluntary accreditation program is carried out by the National League for Nursing and most schools and programs are so accredited.

Diploma Programs. These are typically three-year programs in hospital-based schools of nursing. These schools had their origin in the training schools for nursing that began to be established in the 1870s and that were originally based on the nursing education principles newly established in London by Florence Nightingale.[11] Significant for the future development of nursing education in the United States was the fact that most of these schools were developed as integral parts of hospitals and became closely associated with the provision of hospital nursing services in an essentially apprentice system.

Until recently, the great majority of nursing graduates came from diploma schools. With the increasing development of college programs, the percentage of diploma graduates has declined and the total number of such programs is diminishing. Contributing to the decline in the hospital programs has been the increased costs associated with improved curricula and decreased emphasis on meeting hospital service needs.

Baccalaureate Programs. These are four- or five-year college or university-based programs that lead to the bachelor of science degree. Clinical experience is obtained in university or affiliated teaching hospitals.

11. The first three of these schools in the United States were the Bellevue Training School for Nurses, the Connecticut Training School, and the Massachusetts General Hospital Training School (all established in 1873).

The first school established within a university was at the University of Minnesota (1910). Such schools began to come to prominence in the 1930s and have steadily expanded in numbers; in 1978-79 they graduated 32.5 percent of new nurses.

Associate Degree Programs. These are two-year programs, usually based in junior and community colleges, leading to an associate in arts degree. Practical experience is obtained in affiliated hospitals. Such programs were first established in 1952[12] and have rapidly increased, graduating 47.2 percent of new nurses in 1978-79.

Licensure. The first licensure acts for nurses were passed in 1903, and by 1923 all states and the District of Columbia had such laws. At first, licensure was not mandatory for the practice of nursing; the laws merely prohibited unlicensed persons from using the title "registered nurse." Now all such laws are mandatory, defining and regulating entry to nursing practice. These statutes, called *nursing practice acts* are administered by state nursing boards, variously named Boards of Nursing, Boards of Nursing Examiners, Boards of Nursing Education and Nurse Registration, and so forth. Requirements include a written examination developed by the National Council of State Boards of Nursing. Graduates of diploma, baccalaureate, and associate degree programs take the same examinations given on the same days in all states and all then become registered nurses.

Graduates of foreign nursing schools who meet certain educational and other criteria may take an examination administered abroad by the Commission on Graduates of Foreign Nursing Schools, in conjunction with the Department of Labor and the Immigration and Naturalization Service. Those who pass and are granted the necessary visa are eligible to take state board examinations for U.S. licensure.

Advanced Training and Specialization. There are many *master's degree* programs that have been developed for the advanced training of nurses in nursing education, administration, and clinical special-

---

12. They were established by seven colleges in cooperation with the Cooperative Research Project in Junior and Community College Education, Teachers College, Columbia University.

ties.[13] The clinical specialty programs include public health (community health), medical/surgical, maternal and child health, mental health/psychiatric, cardiovascular, geriatrics/gerontology, and rehabilitation nursing.

Graduates of the clinical specialty programs are often termed *nurse clinicians* or *clinical nurse specialists*. The increasing popularity of educational programs in the clinical specialties is a manifestation of a trend toward making available opportunities for professional advancement for nurses by increasing clinical skills as opposed to the traditional routes of teaching or administration.[14] Other examples are the hospital in-service training programs for nurses in intensive care and coronary care units; and the *nurse practitioner* programs that have been developed for ambulatory care settings (see Chapter 3).

A related development in nursing practice has been the trend toward relieving nurses of non-nursing administrative and clerical tasks so that more of their energy can be devoted to patient care. One manifestation of this trend has been the establishment of *unit manager* positions in many hospitals.

Two older types of nurse specialists are particularly noteworthy: *nurse midwives* and *nurse anesthetists*.

Nurse Anesthetists.   Nurse anesthetists are registered nurses who have received special training in the administration of anesthesia. They have been employed in hospital surgical units since before 1900. The first school for their formal training was established at Lakeside Hospital in Cleveland in about 1910. Programs now are generally of eighteen-months' duration and lead to certification.

Nurse-Midwives.   Nurse-midwives[15] are registered nurses with special training in prenatal and postpartum care and the management

13. Advanced education for professional nurses had its origins in programs established at Teachers College, Columbia University—in a course for those who would be teaching in nursing schools (1900) and courses in public health nursing (1910).

14. For example, the usual route for advancement in hospital nursing has been from staff nurse to head nurse, nursing supervisor, assistant director, and, ultimately, director of nurses.

15. Lay midwives, often called "granny midwives," for many years practiced among poor populations, especially in the rural South. They are licensed in many states, although in many instances no new licenses are being issued. In recent years, in the setting of the woman's health movement, lay midwives are again attending home births in some areas, especially in the West. They are generally not licensed.

of normal labor and delivery. They practice collaboratively with obstetricians.

The first U.S. training school was established in New York City in 1932. Nurse-midwives trained in Britain had been practicing with the Frontier Nursing Service in Kentucky since 1927, and a School of Midwifery was established there in 1939. Programs, leading to certification, are from eight to twenty-four months, the longest leading to a master's degree.

Nurse-midwives are separately licensed in many states. Their legal right to manage normal deliveries (with obstetricians available as needed) has been established by all states.

A number of *doctoral degree* programs in nursing have been established since the mid-1940s. This level of education is being encouraged by many nursing educators for nurses pursuing teaching and research careers in collegiate programs.

National Joint Practice Commission. This commission was established in 1971 by the American Medical Association and the American Nurses' Association and functioned through January 1981. It addressed issues arising from the expanded role of nurses and changing interpretations of "nursing" and "medical" practice. It's activities included the funding in several hospitals of demonstration units for more collaborative nurse–physician practice.[16]

Practical Nurses

Practical nurses are recognized in all states as *licensed practical nurses* (LPNs) or, in California and Texas only, as *licensed vocational nurses* (LVNs).

The first educational programs in practical nursing were established under provisions of the Vocational Education Act of 1917 (Smith–Hughes Act). They are based in vocational and technical schools, hospitals, and community colleges and are generally of eight to fifteen months' duration. Most practical nurses work in hospitals and nursing homes and are under the general, often nominal, supervision of registered nurses.

---

16. See *Guidelines for Establishing Joint or Collaborative Practice in Hospitals* (Chicago: National Joint Practice Commission, 1981).

The licensing agency in most states is the state nursing board; there is a separate board of practical nursing examiners in several states. In about half the states, licensing is mandatory, regulating practice; in the others, it is voluntary, protecting the title.[17]

Nursing Aides (Nursing Assistants)

Nursing aides are important personnel in hospitals and nursing homes. They perform many tasks related to personal care of patients. Education requirements are those specified by the hiring institution, usually some years of high school. Training is on the job with scope, duration, and formality varying greatly among institutions. Nursing aides traditionally have been female. Their male counterparts have traditionally been *orderlies* and *attendants.*

Associations

American Nurses' Association (ANA). This is the professional association for registered nurses and is particularly concerned with nursing practice and the nursing profession. Among its many activities is the certification of nurses in several of the clinical nursing specialties. Many of its constituent state organizations act as collective bargaining agents for nurses.

National League for Nursing (NLN). This association includes agencies, institutions, and individual registered and practical nurses, nursing aides, and other (non-nursing) persons interested in nursing. It is particularly concerned with the improvement of organized nursing services and educational programs. It is the accrediting body for nursing education.

American College of Nurse-Midwives. This is the professional association for nurse-midwives. Its activities include the accreditation of training programs and the certification of their graduates.

American Association of Nurse Anesthetists. This is the professional association for nurse anesthetists. The requirements for membership include a qualifying examination.

17. The term "waivered" practical nurse refers to those who, in certain states, have been licensed on the basis of previous practice, without the educational requirements.

The National Federation of Licensed Practical Nurses. This organization is the professional association for practical nurses.

OTHER PROFESSIONS AND OCCUPATIONS

Medicine and nursing are the two large generalist professions in health care. Other health professions are usually more narrowly focused. Some of these professions are concerned with parts of the body, such as eye care, dentistry and allied professions, and podiatry. The mental health professions focus on a related group of illnesses. Some professions are concerned with specific technologies such as laboratories and x-rays. The public health professions are concerned with the health of populations, rather than individual patients.

Other specialized professions include administration, dietetics and nutrition, health education, medical records, pharmacy, rehabilitation, social work, and veterinary medicine. There are also nonallied groups such as chiropractors, naturopaths, and spiritual healers.

Dentistry and Allied Professions

A minimum of two years of college is required for admission to dental school. About 50 percent of dental students have a bachelor's degree, and this percentage is increasing. Most dental schools require four academic years to obtain the DMD (Doctor of Dental Medicine) or DDS (Doctor of Dental Surgery) degree, although some now have a three calendar year program. For all practical purposes, there is no difference between the DMD and DDS degrees. Dentists and physicians are both doctors, so it is inappropriate to say "dentists and doctors."

To be admitted to dental school one must take the Dental Aptitude Test (DAT) prepared by the Division of Educational Measurements of the American Dental Association (ADA). In the first two years (basic science years) of dental school, in some universities, the dental students take the same courses as medical students, with the addition of oral anatomy, oral pathology, and other preclinical dental science courses. The third and fourth years are usually the clinical years, when students treat patients under faculty supervision in the school's clinics or community facilities. Now some schools are blending the basic sciences and clinical years. Dental internships and residencies are not required for general practice, but are required for board certification in a dental specialty. The eight recognized dental specialties are:

1. Endodontics (root treatment)
2. Oral pathology (the study of diseased oral tissues)
3. Oral surgery
4. Orthodontics (straightening of the teeth)
5. Pedodontics (children's dentistry)
6. Periodontology or Periodontics (treatment of the gums, bone, and other tissues surrounding the teeth)
7. Prosthodontics (replacing missing teeth)
8. Public health dentistry

In addition to the dental degree, all states and the District of Columbia require a written and practical examination for licensure. A certificate from the National Board of Dental Examiners is accepted in place of the written exam in all states except Delaware and Arizona. Regional Dental Examining Boards have been established and successful completion of those examinations is accepted as satisfying the practical examination requirement for several specified states.

Canadian dental education is accepted in most states, but graduates from other foreign dental schools must take the last two clinical years in a U.S. dental school before being examined for licensure. The Science Achievement Examination for Dentistry allows up to two years advance placement in a U.S. dental school.

About 90 percent of active dentists are in private practice and most are in general practice, although specialization is increasing. Other careers include research, teaching, and administration. There is a growing interest in allied dental occupations including:

Dental hygienists require two years of formal education and training as well as state licensure. Dental hygienists work in dental offices specializing in preventive dental care, including the cleaning of teeth and patient education.

Dental assistants assist the dentist in patient care. There are no educational requirements although there are many dental assistant training programs of one or more years. National examination and certification is possible.

Dental laboratory technicians (sometimes called ***denturists***) perform mechanical and technical procedures involved in the fabrication of artificial teeth and dentures. A person may enter this profession with either two years of education or through apprenticeship and on-the-job training. Denturists have been licensed in Oregon to provide dentures directly to the public. Requirements include graduation from a two-year curriculum.

Emerging programs train ***dental therapists, expanded duty auxiliaries***, or ***expanded duty dental assistants (EDDAs)***. This development is similar in concept to physician's assistants. These new personnel undertake a wider range of tasks than dental hygienists, but a smaller range than dentists.

Eye Care

Ophthalmology is the medical specialty and is concerned with medical and surgical care of the eye. Such a physician is an ***ophthalmologist*** or ***eye physician***. An ***optometrist*** has the Doctor of Optometry degree (OD) and is licensed in all states to examine eyes for vision problems, to prescribe and fit glasses but not to perform surgery. A minimum of two years of college is required before the four-year graduate school of optometry. The American Optometric Association estimates that optometrists perform 75 percent of all eye examinations. Two allied occupations are the ***optometric technicians*** and the ***optometric assistant*** who assist ophthalmologists and optometrists. Two-year programs provide education for these occupations. ***Opticians*** dispense eyeglasses prescribed by an ophthalmologist or optometrist. They are high school graduates who have had four to five years of apprenticeship or a one- or two-year training program.

Podiatry

Podiatrists or chiropodists (these terms are synonymous) diagnose and treat (including surgery) disease and deformities of the feet. Schools of podiatry require two years of college before admission, and four years before receiving the DSC (Doctor of Surgical Chiropody) or Pod.D. (Doctor of Podiatry) degree. Internship is optional and not required for state licensure, although examination is. All states license podiatrists. The professional association is the *American Podiatry Association* (APA).

Mental Health

Psychiatry is the medical specialty. Some psychiatrists take further training and undergo psychoanalysis themselves, usually under the auspices of one of several psychoanalytic institutes in order to practice *psychoanalysis*. This is usually a more prolonged form of treatment, often lasting several years, and is built on the ideas of Sigmund Freud.

Psychologists are not physicians but have a master's or Ph.D. degree in psychology. There are several major branches of psychology only one of which, *clinical psychology*, is directly involved in patient care, the others being more academic and research focused. There are several new doctor of psychology degree programs for clinical psychologists. *The American Psychological Association* (APA) defines a professional psychologist (including clinical psychologist, counseling psychologist, school psychologist, and industrial psychologist) as having a doctoral degree from an accredited program. Clinical psychologists use various forms of psychotherapy to treat mental illness but do not prescribe drugs. They work either as independent practitioners or as employees of institutions and organizations providing mental health care. In 1978 all states licensed clinical psychologists with doctoral degrees (but as of 1979 three states had not renewed these laws).

Persons with master's degrees in psychology, counseling, or guidance also provide mental health therapy, usually under the general supervision of psychiatrists or Ph.D. psychologists. A few states license them and five states permit independent unsupervised practice. Licensure is under the titles of psychological associate, psychological examiner, educational psychologist, or school psychologist.[18]

---

18. For a detailed discussion of issues related to psychologists and counselors see *Licensing and Certification of Psychologists and Counselors* by Bruce Fretz and David Mills (San Francisco: Jossey–Bass, 1980).

A major branch of social work concentrates on mental health care. A growing number of states are licensing *psychiatric social workers* who can then provide psychotherapy to their own patients or clients on a fee-for-service basis. *Psychiatric nurses* also work in collaboration with other mental health practitioners and may also provide therapy to their own private patients.

Issues related to the questions of private practice of psychiatrists, clinical psychologists, counselors, and social workers are hotly argued in terms of expertise, types of services provided, and third party reimbursement.

Laboratory Professions

Pathology, microbiology, and *biochemistry* are the medical and biological specialties. There are also a number of types of associated technologists whose professional association is the American Society for Medical Technology.

Medical Technologists require three years of college and one year in one of about 800 approved training schools. Afterwards, passing the examination confers the title MT (ASCP). ASCP stands for the American Society for Clinical Pathologists, which helps administer the exam.

Cytotechnologists require two years of college, six months in an approved program, and six months' experience in an acceptable laboratory. After this, passing the certifying exam allows one to use the designation CT (ASCP). Cytology (in this context) is the detection of certain cellular changes, especially precancerous or cancerous changes.[19]

Blood Bank Technologists are registered medical technologists who have had an additional year's training in a blood bank school approved by the American Association of Blood Banks. The examination confers the title MT (ASCP) BB.

Histologic Technicians prepare sections of body tissues for microscopic examination. They require a year of supervised training in a

---

19. This technique was developed by George Papanicolaou, hence the well-known "Pap" test for detection of cancer of the female reproductive system.

clinical pathology laboratory, beyond high school. Examination confers certification as HT (ASCP).

Certified Laboratory Assistants work under the supervision of medical technologists. It requires one year of hospital training beyond high school, and passing an examination confers the letters CLA.

Radiology

Radiology is the medical specialty. *Radiologic technologists* (also called *x-ray technicians*) assist the radiologist. Various forms of training are possible, including a twenty-four-month program in an approved hospital-based school. Some of these programs extend over a four-year period and entitle the graduate to the degree of bachelor of science in x-ray technology. The hospital schools usually charge no tuition and have two to six students, on average. *Nuclear medical technologists* have an MT (ASCP) or a BS degree in biologic or chemical sciences, plus a year's training. They may work in radiology or laboratory settings.

Public Health

Public health is concerned with preventing disease through population-based programs rather than the medical care of individual patients. These are largely government-based services at the federal, state, or local level. University-based schools of public health provide education in a variety of areas including:

Environmental health (air pollution control, accident prevention, occupational medicine, industrial safety, control of radiological hazards, sewage and solid waste disposal, sanitation engineering, provision of clean water supplies, and fluoridation)

Population studies (family planning, population control)

Demography (the study of population size, distribution, and characteristics)

Biostatistics (the application of statistics to health problems)

Nutrition (the relationship between food use and production, and health)

Infectious diseases (including tropical public health)

Epidemiology (the study of the impact of disease on populations)

Maternal and child health

Public health nursing

Public health dentistry

Public health education

Health services administration (medical care administration)

The national organization is the American Public Health Association.

Administration (Health Administration, Hospital Administration, Health Management)

Educational programs in health services administration are located in schools of public health, business schools, schools of government or public administration, medical schools, or in a combination of the above. Courses and degrees are provided at the baccalaureate, master, and doctorate levels. The *Association of University Programs in Health Administration* (AUPHA) is a voluntary organization that represents most of these programs.

Dietetics and Nutrition

Dieticians specialize in feeding people, and their profession is largely hospital based. They can specialize in teaching, research, administration, and therapy (planning special menus and diets). The *nutritionist* is, in practice, an educator who often works in a public health setting. Both professions require a college education. Master and doctorate degrees are available. Dieticians ordinarily take a one-year internship, and postcollege education is recommended for nutritionists. *The American Dietetic Association* (ADA) serves as the professional association for both groups. The dietician brings knowledge of, and skills in, nutrition and management to the feeding of individuals and groups. The nutritionist is concerned with carrying out nutritional programs for the promotion of health and prevention of disease, consults with other professionals, and provides education for both health professionals and the public.

Health Education

Health educators work with individuals and communities, teaching and promoting good health practices. There are bachelor's degree programs for both *school health educators* and *public health (community health) educators.* School health educators work in elementary and secondary schools and must meet state certification requirements for teachers. Public health educators work in health departments, voluntary agencies, hospitals and ambulatory care programs. A master's degree is required for some health education positions. The professional associations are the *American School Health Association* and the *Society for Public Health Education.*

Medical Record Administration

Medical record administrators are concerned with storing and retrieving information about patients' past health status and care. Traditionally a central concern of this profession has been the management of medical record departments in hospitals. Computerization of medical information is transforming such information systems. There are baccalaureate degree programs in *medical record administration*, and two-year associate degree programs for *medical record technicians.* Graduates passing a national exam can become a *registered record administrator (RRA)* or an *accredited record technician (ART).* The national association is the *American Medical Record Association.*

Pharmacy

Pharmacy is an applied physical and biological science: the practice of preparing, preserving, and dispensing therapeutic drugs. For many pharmacists it combines a professional and business career. About 80 percent of all pharmacists are in retail or community pharmacy. (See Chapter 9.) Some of these drugstores limit themselves to health products, while others sell a wide range of products. About 10 percent of pharmacists work in hospital-based pharmacies. The remainder work in industry, government, or teaching.

Pharmacy requires five years of education after high school for a BS in pharmacy. Prior to 1960, four years were required. Of the current five years, the first two are preprofessional (liberal arts) and the last three are professional. Transfer students are accepted from junior colleges or liberal arts schools. The three professional years include the study of pharmaceutical chemistry, pharmacognosy (the study of natural drugs from plants and animals), pharmacology (the action of drugs in the body), toxicology (the effects of poisons on the body, and antidotes), pharmacy administration, and clinical pharmacy. Master's and doctoral degrees of pharmacy are also awarded. Licensure ordinarily requires a degree from an accredited school; an apprenticeship or internship of six months to one year under the supervision of a licensed pharmacist; and passage of the state board examination. The professional society is the *American Pharmaceutical Association.*

Rehabilitation

The medical specialty is physical medicine and rehabilitation (physiatry).

Physical therapy is concerned with the restoration of function and prevention of disability following disease or injury. Qualifications can be obtained in three ways: (1) a four-year bachelor's degree program; (2) a twelve-month certificate course for people with a bachelor's degree; and (3) master's degree training. Physical therapists are licensed.

Occupational therapy requires four years of college leading to a bachelor of science in occupational therapy. In addition, nine to ten months of clinical training is required. There is also an optional additional eighteen months of academic and clinical training for advanced standing, and some master's degree programs. Those who pass the national registration exam may use the designation OTR. These therapists specialize in the maintenance and restoration of function, especially through manual activities. *Occupational therapy assistants* require high school graduation plus a training program. The *prosthetist* makes and fits artificial limbs and the *orthotist* makes and fits orthopedic braces, both working from a physician's prescription. Professional associations include the *American Physical Therapy Association*, the *American Occupational Therapy Association* and the *American Academy of Orthotists and Prosthetists.*

Social Work

Two years of graduate education in a school of social work lead to the Master of Social Work (MSW) degree. The curriculum combines classroom instruction and field experience covering social welfare policy and services, human behavior, social environment, and social work practice. Areas of concentration include service to individuals (social case work), groups (social group work), and communities (community organization), and administration, research, and social policy. There are also four-year bachelor's degree programs in social work whose graduates are also considered professional social workers.

Social workers practice both inside the health field and in other areas. Major practice settings include health, mental health, child welfare, family services, aging, juvenile and adult justice, and community service and planning. The professional association is the *National Association of Social Workers* (NASW).

Veterinary Medicine

Veterinarians receive the DVM (or VMD) degree. Most veterinarians are in private practice. The work of veterinarians affects human health because veterinarians are involved in research on animals that has application to human medicine. There are diseases that are transmitted from animals to man, and the health of cattle, sheep, and other animals is important because these animals are sources of human food. The professional society is the *American Vetinary Medicine Association.*

Nonallied Groups

Chiropractic is a system of mechanical therapeutics based on the principle that the nervous system largely determines the state of health. Treatment consists primarily of chiropractic manipulation, usually of the spinal column. Some chiropractors ("mixers" as opposed to "straights"), also use physiotherapy and dietary modification and radiology for diagnosis. Drugs and surgery are not used. There are about 20,000 licensed chiropractors, mostly in California, New York, Texas, Missouri, and Pennsylvania. Licensure usually requires the completion of two years of college, and then a four-year chiropractic course leading to the degree of Doctor of Chiropractic (DC). The national association is the *American Chiropractic Association.*

Naturopaths rely on the natural healing processes and natural remedies such as special foods and diets, massage, and heat.

Spiritual healers (faith healers) use the power of religious faith to cure illness. For example, Christian Science, founded in the last century by Mary Baker Eddy and based in Boston, Massachusetts, does not accept the idea that medicine can cure illness; only the Deity can. There are Christian Science practitioners and nurses who provide spiritual help, advice, and physical assistance to the ill at home, and in Christian Science nursing homes and sanitoria. The Indian Health Service has encouraged some use of Navaho native faith healers as intermediaries between the Navaho Indians and modern medicine, in order to maintain Navaho tribal customs and the benefits of their healing ceremonies.

Curanderas (healers) play a large role in some American Hispanic communities. Without formal training, using traditional theories of illness and treatment, they provide herbal remedies and counseling. The psychological support they provide is consistent with their patients' cultural traditions—a feature often missing in American medical care.

LABOR UNIONS

The activities of American labor unions are prescribed in great detail by federal laws, court decisions, and the administrative rulings of the National Labor Relations Board (NLRB), an agency of the federal government. The important federal labor laws are The Wagner Act of 1935 and the Taft–Hartley Act of 1947 (the National Labor Relations Act and amendments). These laws define rights and obligations of unions and employers with respect to fair labor practices and collective bargaining. Originally nonprofit hospitals were excluded from these acts. This was changed by the 1974 Nonprofit Hospital Amendments (PL93-360). As a result, unionization of health workers has been growing.

Unionization. A group of workers may choose to have an election by secret ballot to decide if they wish to be represented in collective bargaining by a union. Workers are defined as a bargaining group that may include all or part of the workers in an organization. There are many different unions representing health workers throughout the country.

Unionization of Professionals. Nurses and staff physicians have become unionized in some organizations. Some medical residents have organized into unions but are considered students by the NLRB and therefore do not have legal support for collective bargaining. In some cases statewide professional associations, such as state nursing associations, have become qualified as a union, and bargain collectively for their membership.

American unions, unlike many foreign unions, focus narrowly on pay, fringe benefits, and working conditions, rather than creating political parties or striving for wide-ranging social objectives.

Labor unions for workers in general play an important role in health care through collective bargaining for health insurance benefits with employers. For example, the United Automobile Workers based in Detroit has been very active in efforts to improve and provide medical care for their members. Some labor unions have created medical care delivery systems, including health maintenance organizations. Large health employers have played similar roles, often in cooperation with their employees' unions.

SELECTED READINGS

Job Descriptions and Organizational Analysis for Hospitals and Related Health Services, rev. ed. (Washington, D.C.: U.S. Government Printing Office, 1971).

American Medicine and the Public Interest, Rosemary Stevens (New Haven: Yale University Press, 1971).

The Advance of American Nursing, Philip and Beatrice Kalisch (Boston: Little Brown, 1978).

Facts about Nursing: A Statistical Summary. Published periodically by the American Nurses' Association.

Table 4-1.   List of Health Occupations.

Type of Work Primary Title	Relevant and Some Alternative Titles
Administration	Hospital Administrator Nursing Home Administrator Clinic Manager Health Officer, Medical Care Administrator Health Planner Health Program Analyst
Anthropology and Sociology	Medical Anthropologist, Medical Sociologist
Automatic Data Processing	Computer Operator, Systems Analyst
Basic Sciences in the Health Field	Scientist Ecologist Anatomist Epidemiologist Biologist Microbiologist Botanist Pharmacologist Chemist
Biomedical Engineering	
Chiropractic	
Clinical Laboratory Service	Clinical Laboratory, Scientists, Technicians, and Technologists
Dentistry and Allied Services	Dentist, Dental Hygienist, Dental Assistant, Dental Laboratory Technician
Dietetic and Nutritional Service	Dietetic Assistant Food Service Manager Dietitian Food Service Worker Nutritionist
Economic Research in the Health Field	Medical Economist
Environmental Sanitation	Environmental Technologist Food, Milk, Sanitarian
Food and Drug Protective Service	Food and Drug Chemist or Microbiologist, or Inspector Health Inspector
Health and Vital Statistics	Demographer Biomathematician Health Statistician Vital Record Registrar
Health Education	Health Educator
Health Information and Communication	Biomedical Photographer Medical Illustrator Medical Writer
Library Services in the Health Field	Medical Librarian Medical Library Assistant
Medical Records	Medical Record Administrator or Librarian or Technologist or Aide, or Technician

Table 4-1. continued

Type of Work Primary Title	Relevant and Some Alternative Titles
Medicine and Osteopathy	(See List of Medical Specialties)
Midwifery	Nurse Midwife
Nursing and Related Services	Registered Nurse Licensed Practical Nurse Home Health Aide Attendant Nursing Aide Orderly
Occupational Therapy	Occupational Therapist Occupational Therapy Aide Occupational Therapy Assistant
Opticianry	Dispensing Optician Optical Mechanic
Optometry	Optometrist Optometric Assistant, Technician Vision Care Aide, Technologist
Orthotic and Prosthetic Technology	Orthotist (Orthopedic Brace Maker) Prosthetist (Prosthetic Appliance Maker)
Pharmacy	Pharmacist Pharmacy Aide, Assistant, Technician
Physical Therapy	Physical Therapist Physical Therapist Aide, Assistant
Podiatric Medicine	Podiatrist (Chiropodist)
Psychology	Phychologist (Clinical, Counseling, Developmental, School, Social)
Radiologic Technology	Nuclear Medicine, Radiation Therapy, Technician Radiologic Technician
Respiratory Therapy	Respiratory Therapist, Aide Technician (Inhalation Therapist)
Secretarial and Office Services	Dental, Medical Secretary, Receptionist, Office Assistant
Social Work	Social Worker (Caseworker), Social Work Assistant, Technician
Special Rehabilitation Service	Rehabilitation Specialist Music, Recreation Therapists
Speech Pathology and Audiology	Audiologist, Speech Pathologist
Veterinary Medicine	Veterinarian
Vocational Rehabilitation Counseling	Vocational Rehabilitation Counselor

(Table 4-1. continued overleaf)

Table 4-1. continued

Type of Work *Primary Title*	*Relevant and Some Alternative Titles*
Miscellaneous Health Services	
Animal Technician	
Cardiopulmonary Technician	
Community Health Aide	
Electrocardiograph Technician	
Electroencephalograph Technician	
Emergency Medical Technician	
(Ambulance Aide, Attendant, Driver)	
Extracorporeal Circulation Specialist	
Medical Assistant	
Operating Room Technician	
Ophthalmic Assistant	
Orthoptist	
Physician's Assistant	
(MEDEX, Clinical Associate,	
Community Health Medic)	

Source: *Health Resources Statistics, 1974.* National Center for Health Statistics, U.S. Department of Health, Education and Welfare, Public Health Service, (Rockville, Maryland), 1974, pp. 517-533.

Table 4-2. Persons 16 Years of Age and Over Employed in Selected Health-Related Occupations: United States, Selected Years 1970-79. (*Data are based on household interviews of a sample of the civilian noninstitutionalized population*).

Occupation	Year					
	1970[a]	1975	1976	1977	1978	1979
	Number of Persons in Thousands					
Total, 16 years and over	3,103	4,169	4,341	4,517	4,753	4,951
Physicians, medical and osteopathic	281	354	368	403	424	431
Dentists	91	110	107	105	117	131
Pharmacists	110	119	123	138	136	135
Registered nurses	830	935	999	1,063	1,112	1,223
Therapists	75	157	159	178	189	207
Health technologists and technicians	260	397	436	462	498	534
Health administrators	84	152	162	175	184	185
Dental assistants	88	126	122	123	130	134
Health aides, excluding nursing	119	211	229	234	270	281
Nursing aides, orderlies, and attendants	718	1,001	1,002	1,008	1,037	1,024
Practical nurses	237	370	381	371	402	376
Other health-related occupations[b]	210	237	253	257	254	290

a. Based on the 1970 decennial census; all other years are annual averages derived from the Current Population Survey.

b. Includes chiropractors, optometrists, podiatrists, veterinarians, dietitians, embalmers, funeral directors, opticians, lens grinders and polishers, dental lab technicians, lay midwives, and health trainees.

Note: Data were compiled by the U.S. Bureau of the Census from the Current Population Survey. These data differ from those published by the National Center for Health Statistics in various editions of *Health Resources Statistics*, because the latter are derived from a variety of sources.

Source: U.S. Department of Health and Human Services, *Health United States 1980*, Public Health Service (Washington, D.C.: U.S. Government Printing Office, 1980), p. 187.

Table 4-3. Persons Employed in the Health Service Industry, According to Place of Employment: United States, 1970-79 (*Data are based on household interviews of a sample of the civilian noninstitutionalized population*).

Place of Employment	Year		
	1970[a]	1975	1979
	Number of Persons in Thousands		
Total	*4,247*	*5,865*	*6,849*
Office of physicians	477	607	755
Office of dentists	222	327	385
Hospitals	2,690	3,394	3,843
Convalescent institutions	509	884	1,035
Office of other health practitioners	61	90	84
Other health service sites	288	563	747

a. April 1, derived from decennial census; all other data years are July 1 estimates.

Note: Totals exclude persons in health-related occupations who are working in non-health industries, as classified by the U.S. Bureau of the Census, such as pharmacists employed in drug-stores, school nurses, and nurses working in private households.

Source: U.S. Department of Health and Human Services, *Health United States 1980*, Public Health Service (Washington, D.C.: U.S. Government Printing Office, 1980), p. 186. (U.S. Bureau of the Census and U.S. Bureau of Labor Statistics.)

Table 4-4. Accrediting Agencies for Selected Educational Programs.

Educational Program	Accrediting Agencies[a]
Blood Bank Technology	1. Committee on Allied Health Education and Accreditation (CAHEA) of the American Medical Association (AMA) 2. American Association of Blood Banks
Cytotechnology	1. CAHEA 2. American Society of Clinical Pathologists (ASCP)
Dental Hygiene Dentistry	Commission on Dental Accreditation, American Dental Association
Dietetics	Commission on Accreditation, American Dietetic Association
Emergency Medical Technology	1. CAHEA 2. American College of Emergency Physicians 3. American College of Surgeons 4. American Psychiatric Association 5. American Society of Anesthesiologists 6. National Association of Emergency Medical Technicians 7. National Registry of Emergency Medical Technicians
Health Services Administration (Graduate Programs)	Accrediting Commission on Education for Health Services Administration
Medical Assistants	1. CAHEA 2. American Association of Medical Assistants
Medical Records	1. CAHEA 2. American Medical Record Association
Medical Technology	1. CAHEA 2. American Society for Medical Technology 3. American Society for Microbiology 4. ASCP
Medicine	Liaison Committee on Medical Education; Joint Committee of the Association of American Medical Colleges, AMA and Canadian Medical Association
Nuclear Medicine Technology	1. CAHEA 2. American College of Radiology 3. American Society for Medical Technology 4. ASCP 5. American Society of Radiologic Technologists 6. Society of Nuclear Medicine
Occupational Therapy	1. CAHEA 2. American Occupational Therapy Association
Osteopathic Medicine	American Osteopathic Association
Pharmacy	American Council on Pharmaceutical Education

Table 4-4. continued

Physical Therapy	1. CAHEA 2. American Academy of Physical Medicine and Rehabilitation 3. American Academy of Neurology
Physician's Assistant 　Assistant to primary care 　　physicians 　Surgeon's assistant	1. CAHEA 2. American Academy of Family Physicians 3. American Academy of Physician's Assistants 4. American College of Physicians 5. American College of Surgeons 6. American Society of Internal Medicine 7. Association of Physician Assistant Programs
Podiatry	American Podiatry Association
Practical Nursing	1. National League for Nursing 2. National Association for Practical Nurse Education and Service
Professional Nursing	National League for Nursing
Public Health	Council on Education for Public Health
Radiologic Technology	1. CAHEA 2. American College of Radiology 3. American Society of Radiologic Technologists
Respiratory Therapy	1. CAHEA 2. American Association for Respiratory Therapy 3. American College of Chest Physicians 4. American Society of Anesthesiologists 5. American Thoracic Society
Social Work	Council on Social Work Education
Speech Pathology and Audiology	American Speech, Language, and Hearing Association

a. Numbered agencies mean there is a joint accreditation program.

Sources: "Annual Report on Medical Education in the United States 1979-1980," *Journal of the American Medical Association* 244 (1980): 2838; Sherry S. Harris, ed., *Accredited Institutions of Postsecondary Education 1980-81*, published for the Council on Postsecondary Accreditation by the American Council on Education (Washington, D.C.: 1980).

Table 4-5. Professionally Active Physicians (MDs), According to Primary Specialty: United States, Selected Years 1970, 1975, and 1978 (*Data are based on reporting by physicians*).

	Year		
Primary Specialty	1970	1975	1978
	Number of Physicians		
Professionally active physicians	304,926	335,608	371,343
Primary care	115,505	128,745	141,610
General practice[a]	56,804	53,714	55,414
Internal medicine	41,196	53,712	62,056
Pediatrics	17,505	21,319	24,140
Other medical specialties	17,127	18,743	22,277
Dermatology	3,937	4,594	5,032
Pediatric allergy	388	439	431
Pediatric cardiology	471	527	575
Internal medicine subspecialties[b]	12,331	13,183	16,239
Surgical specialties	84,545	94,776	101,216
General surgery	29,216	31,173	31,699
Neurological surgery	2,537	2,898	3,071
Obstetrics and gynecology	18,498	21,330	23,591
Ophthalmology	9,793	11,011	11,798
Orthopedic surgery	9,467	11,267	12,553
Otolaryngology	5,305	5,670	6,040
Plastic surgery	1,583	2,224	2,610
Colon and rectal surgery	663	655	673
Thoracic surgery	1,779	1,960	2,025
Urology	5,704	6,588	7,156
Other specialties	87,749	93,344	106,240
Anesthesiology	10,725	12,741	14,137
Neurology	3,027	4,085	4,873
Pathology	10,135	11,603	12,517
Forensic pathology	193	186	232
Psychiatry	20,901	23,683	25,379
Child psychiatry	2,067	2,557	2,897
Physical medicine and rehabilitation	1,443	1,615	1,851
Radiology	10,380	11,417	11,495
Diagnostic radiology	1,941	3,500	5,388
Therapeutic radiology	855	1,161	1,389
Miscellaneous[c]	26,082	20,796	26,082

a. Includes general practice and family practice.

b. Includes gastroenterology, pulmonary diseases, allergy, and cardiovascular diseases.

c. Includes occupational medicine, general preventive medicine, aerospace medicine, public health, other specialties not listed, and unspecified specialties.

Note: Active Federal and non-Federal doctors of medicine (MDs) in the fifty states and the District of Columbia are included. Physicians not classified, inactive physicians, and physicians with unknown address in the United States are excluded. For 1978, this includes 25,102 physicians not classified, 26,698 physicians inactive, and 9,291 physicians with unknown address.

Notes to Table 4-5. continued

Source: U.S. Department of Health and Human Services, *Health United States 1980*, Public Health Service (Washington, D.C.: U.S. Government Printing Office, 1980).

5 PAYING FOR CARE

One of the unique features of medical care in the United States is the complexity of its financing. Some care is paid for directly by patients themselves, an increasing proportion is paid for indirectly through a variety of insurance or prepayment plans, and some is provided free of charge to the patient.

Self pay, direct pay, or *out-of-pocket payment* are terms used interchangeably for payment by the patient. In 1978 this accounted for an estimated $55 billion out of $168 billion for total health expenditures. Direct pay covers the majority of payments for dentists, drugs, eyeglasses, and appliances. This category also includes the deductible and coinsurance payments associated with insurance.

Indirect payment includes *health insurance* (sometimes called *prepayment*). A special category is the *health maintenance organization* (HMO), which combines an insurance mechanism with provision of services through either prepaid group practices (PGPs) or individual practice associations (IPAs). Insurance (or prepayment) can be divided into governmental programs like Medicare and Medicaid (see Chapter 6),[1] and nongovernment or private programs. Private insurance includes the nonprofit Blue Cross–Shield plans and

1. Whether Medicaid is in fact a form of health insurance is arguable since it is more simply a system of payments to providers of care on behalf of certain low-income persons. It is more generally considered a part of the public assistance system.

commercial insurance companies. Some large corporations provide their own insurance for their employees using an agent to pay bills and help keep track of the paperwork.

The provision of services without charge is now done mostly by government at the federal, state, or local level to certain eligible populations. Examples are the Veterans Administration medical care system, the Indian Health Service, the health services for the armed forces, state hospitals for mental illness, and some county and municipal hospitals. These are financed by annual budgets derived from tax revenues. (The medical care of the indigent provided by county and municipal hospitals is now paid for in part by the federal and state governments under Medicaid.)

Some free care continues to be given by many nongovernmental hospitals and physicians, although this has diminished with the advent of Medicare and Medicaid. Sometimes this care is truly without charge, sometimes it may be in the form of writing off uncollectable debts. Hospitals that have received federal funds through the Hill–Burton program are also required to give a certain percentage of free care.

HEALTH INSURANCE

Health insurance "carriers" include insurance companies, Blue Cross–Blue Shield, and the Medicare system. (Medicaid is a public assistance program managed by the states.) Medicare and Medicaid are covered in Chapter 6.

Insurance can be defined as protection by written contract against the hazards (in whole or in part) of the happenings of specified fortuitous events.[2] *Health insurance* can be defined as protection against the costs of hospital and medical care of lost income arising from an illness or injury.

Individuals make a contractual agreement, either singly or in groups, with an insurer who promises to pay for an agreed upon range of services under specified conditions. The insurer can pay money directly to the subscriber, or to the provider of services (e.g., Blue Cross–Blue Shield).

2. The source for many of these definitions is *Source Book of Health Insurance Data* (Washington, D.C.: Health Insurance Institute, yearly).

Health insurance requires careful specification of risks to be covered so that insurers can estimate the probable size of their benefit payments. It also is subject to such problems as overutilization of services. If a self-pay patient uses a great many health services, it is only that patient's concern. If other members of an insured group use a great many services, it increases each member's premium payments and, therefore, each member is affected by the behavior of others (a phenomenon economists call *externalities*). In contrast, the direct provision of services has a more controllable and predictable budgeted level of expenditure.

Health Insurance and Prepayment

These terms are used synonymously by many, but others make a distinction between them. The historical reason for such differentiation lies, in part, with the competition between Blue Cross–Blue Shield and insurance companies. Blue Cross enabling legislation was put forward with the argument of their uniqueness summed up in the word "prepayment." Sometimes, insurance companies have argued, these state laws provide unfair competitive advantages to Blue Cross–Blue Shield. They argue that Blue Cross–Blue Shield provides insurance and should be viewed in the same fashion as insurance companies. According to this view, Blue Cross–Blue Shield organizations are nonprofit insurance companies.

The term prepayment has also come to be used synonymously with *capitation payment*—the payment to providers of a fixed monthly fee on behalf of insured persons whether or not services are rendered. Hence, a *prepaid group practice* is a group practice that is paid in this manner, usually by participation in a health maintenance organization.

Some would call most health insurance "prepayment" since it can be argued that many of the services covered will be required with a high degree of probability and thus are not really rare and fortuitous events. This semantic problem is well summarized by McCarthy:

> Health care utilization is not a rare occurrence. On the average, each person in the United States visits a physician five times a year. One out of every seven Americans is admitted to a hospital at least once a year. Other than coverage for catastrophic illness, a fairly rare event, health insurance has become a mechanism for offsetting expected rather than unexpected costs. The

experience of the many is pooled in an effort to reduce expected outlays to manageable prepayment size. Perhaps the term "assurance" more appropriately describes this health care payment system that has evolved. In Britain, "assurance" is used to denote coverage for contingencies that must eventually happen (life assurance); "insurance" is reserved for coverage of those contingencies like fire and theft, which may not occur.[3]

In the health field, the distinction between health insurance and prepayment is probably not a useful one. In practice, all plans that involve a pooling of risks by some sort of advance payment or premium are considered forms of health insurance.

Basic Characteristics of Health Insurance Policies

Coverage —types of illness, types of treatment for which the policyholder will be recompensed (covered).

Age Limits —both for new applicants and renewals.

Exclusions —specified hazards or conditions for which a policy will not provide benefits payments.

Benefits —the amount of money paid for a type of illness or treatment.

> *Service benefits* pay the provider of care for the specific hospital or medical care services rendered. This is done by Blue Cross and Medicare, which have contractual agreements with providers of care, defining appropriate costs and or charges for services provided.

> *Indemnity benefits* pay the insured in the event of a covered loss (for example, $250 a day in the hospital regardless of the actual bill; the actual bill, if deemed reasonable; or in the case of disability insurance, $50 a day for a day lost from work due to illness).

Policy Term —time period covered by the policy.

Pre-existing conditions —physical and/or mental conditions of the insured person that exist prior to the issuance of his or her policy. These may or may not be covered.

Grace Period —a specified time after a policy's premium payment is due in which the protection of the policy continues subject to actual receipt of premium within that time.

3. Carol McCarthy, "Financing for Health Care," in Steven Jonas and contributors, *Health Care Delivery in the United States*, 2nd edition (New York: Springer Publishing Co., 1981), p. 283.

Rider—an amendment to the policy expanding or decreasing benefits.

Time Limit—the period of time in which notice of claim or proof of loss must be filed in order to obtain benefits.

Upper Limit of Coverage—limit set in the policy for maximum payment.

Waiver—an agreement attached to a policy that exempts from coverage certain disabilities normally covered by the policy. (An example would be an injury associated with an unusual and risky activity or for a prior medical condition.)

Hypothetical Example of a Health Insurance Policy. A hospital insurance policy (*coverage*) for people under age sixty-five (*age limit*) pays $100 per day (*benefits*) for each day in the hospital up to fifty days (*upper limit of coverage*). The policy is good for one year (*policy term*) and excludes treatment for mental illness and tuberculosis (*exclusions*). Pre-existing medical conditions are not covered (*pre-existing conditions*), prepayments are due monthly by the fifth day of the month (five-day *grace period*), and the company must receive notice of hospitalization not less than thirty days after admission to the hospital (*time limit*).

More Characteristics of Health Insurance Policies

Premium—The periodic payment required to keep the policy in force.

Claim—A demand by an insured person for benefits provided by a policy; a request for payment.

Noncancellable (Guaranteed Renewable) Policy—(This is the opposite of an "optional renewable policy.") A policy that the insured has the right to continue in force by the timely payment of premiums set forth in the policy to a specified age during which period the insurer has no right to make any change in any provision of the policy while the policy is in force. Usually, the insurer can not change the premium rate for an individual insured person. The insurer may or may not be allowed to make premium rate changes for all similar policyholders.

Group Insurance (as distinct from *individual* or *personal insurance*)— A policy protecting a group of persons, usually employees for a firm, rather than a policy providing protection to a specific policyholder and/or family. One difference is that the insurer estimates the expected risk for the group as a whole, rather than for each individual.

Coinsurance — A policy provision by which both the insured person and the insurance company share the expenses of illness or injury in a specified proportion. (For example, the insurer will pay 80 percent of the hospital bill while the insured pays the remaining 20 percent.)

Deductible — That portion of covered hospital and medical charges that the insured person must pay before benefits begin. This is in contrast to *first dollar coverage*, where there is no deductible.

Assignment of Benefits — Frequently hospitals or other providers of care will have patients assign (transfer) the benefits (indemnity benefits) from the patient to the hospital so that the insurance company pays the hospital directly.

Experience Rating — Individuals or groups are charged premiums proportional to their expected level of utilization.

Community Rating — All the people in a population, regardless of their different risks of becoming ill are charged the same monthly premium. Community rating has been advocated as a way to promote widespread and affordable health insurance coverage and has traditionally been a feature of Blue Cross – Blue Shield plans. In effect it redistributes the costs of medical care from the poorer to the richer, from the old to the young, from large families to small families, from the less to the more healthy. Under competitive conditions, community rating is not possible because other insurors will offer lower premiums to low risk groups. Due to such competitive pressure Blue Cross – Blue Shield has made increasing use of experience rating.

Multiple Coverage — This is when an individual has more than one insurance policy covering the same event.

Hypothetical Example of Deductible, Coinsurance, Upper Limit, and Not Covered Expenses. The hospital bill is $1,000. The insurance policy has a $50 deductible, 10 percent coinsurance and an upper limit of $850. Fifty dollars of the hospital bill is not covered because of exclusions in the policy (uninsured expenses). Diagrammatically this can be represented as shown in Figure 5–1.[4]

---

4. Figures are chosen for ease of calculation, not as typical of policies in use.

Figure 5-1.   An Example of Deductible, Coinsurance, Upper Limit, and Not Covered Expenses.

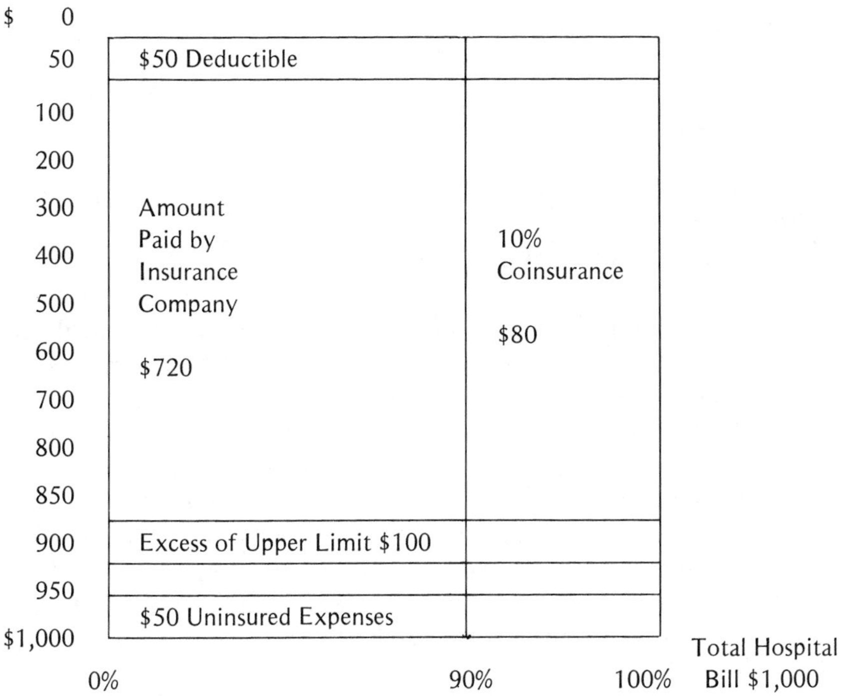

$$total\ bill\ -\ uninsured\ expenses\ =\ \$950$$
$$(\$1,000)\qquad\qquad(\$50)$$

First method of calculation:

$950 - $850 (*upper limit of coverage*) = $100 in excess of upper limit

$850 - $ 50 (*deductible*) = $800.

To which the 10 percent coinsurance feature is applied so that the insurance company pays $720.

The patient pays $50 deductible plus $100 excess over upper limit plus $50 uninsured expenses and $80 coinsurance for a total of $280.[5]

Second method of calculation:

$950 less 10 percent coinsurance ($95) less $50 deductible. The insurance company pays $805.

Third method of calculation:

Remove the $50 deductible first.
Coinsurance is $90.
The insurance company pays $810.

Hypothetical Simplified Example of How Premiums are Calculated. Assume the policy is to pay $100 per day (*benefit*) for each day of hospital care (*coverage*) for the first 50 days for each admission (*upper limit*) for the coming year (*policy term*). It is to cover the 1,000 employees of X Company. The company will pay half the cost and the employees will have the other half deducted from their monthly paychecks. By analyzing the previous year's experience of these employees it was found that the average employee used 1.1 hospital days per year, or 1,100 total days for all 1,000 employees. It was also found that the total number of hospital days in excess of the 50 limit was 100 days.

This leaves 1,000 days of hospital care to be covered at $100 per day, or $100,000 yearly in total benefits. To this figure is added 20 percent for administrative expenses, overhead, reserves, profits, and so forth, for a total needed revenue of $120,000 per year. Of this the company pays half, $60,000, and each individual employee pays $60 per year or $5 per month (the monthly *premium*). Modifications in the benefits would make these calculations much more complex. This kind of analysis is carried out by insurance *actuaries*.

---

5. Note that if the deductions and coinsurance are removed in a different order, the insurance coverage will vary accordingly. The order of calculation would be defined by the policy.

Major Forms of Health Insurance

- Hospital (pays hospital bills).
- Surgical (pays for doctor's operating fees and related care).
- Regular Medical (pays for nonsurgical doctor fees in hospital and for nonhospital physician care).
- Major Medical (pays for all expenses with coinsurance and deductible, designed especially to cover major illness).
  Recent legislative proposals for a national *catastrophic* health insurance are similar to the major medical idea in that they would have large deductibles and pay for the high costs of major illness.
- Disability (loss of income).

Characteristics of an Insured Event

A major problem for insurers and providers is to make their obligations both predictable and bounded by some upper known limit. The actuaries who design insurance plans consider the following ideal characteristics of the event to be covered. These characteristics play a basic role in defining the extent and type of coverage.

- The insured event should be *unpredictable* or random in the individual case but predictable on average. For example, one cannot predict whether an individual coin toss will come up heads or not, but one does know that there is a 50 percent chance of this happening over many tosses. Thus, the concept of pooling of risks. If the event were predictable, then one would buy insurance on the day of the event and let the policy lapse the day after (for example, maternity benefits for already pregnant mothers).
- The insured event should be *definable* so that everyone can agree that it has occurred. For example, a broken leg is definable, but it is not so easy to say when a neurosis calls for psychotherapy.
- The insured event should be *uncontrollable*, like lightning striking a barn.

- The insured event should be relatively *large* so that the administrative costs of writing the insurance coverage are proportionally small. People who can pay for health insurance usually have enough money available to cover low cost events. It is the big costs that may bankrupt them. One reason for deductibles is to avoid the administrative costs of processing small claims.

- Insured events should be *independent* events in the statistical sense. Nonindependent events are the plague, war, and widespread natural disasters where, if one person is harmed, many others will also be harmed. The large expenditures that would result could bankrupt the insurance company.

- Expenses connected with the event should be *finite*, that is, known and limited. This allows insurers to estimate how much they can expect to pay out, and that payments will not be infinitely large. One reason health insurance policies have upper limits is to limit and make finite the size of their payment. This protects, for example, against exorbitant or inflated bills.

- The average predicted probability of the insured event occurring shoud be small enough so that the required premium is affordable. For example, if 95-year-old men who have already had two heart attacks were insured for $100,000 and they have a 50 percent chance of dying within the year, the premium would be prohibitive—$50,000 for that year. No one could afford this kind of insurance.

The more the event is as described above the more appropriate is insurance as a payment mechanism. Medical care does not always fit these characteristics. Chronic disease and annual dental hygiene care are predictable. Medical care costs can vary substantially for the same medical condition and the use of medical care varies substantially from one place and setting to another.

In short, insurance is the pooling of risks and the averaging of their costs. When insurance companies underwrite (cover) a risk they need predictable limits on their commitments. *Reinsurance* is a method of insuring the insurance company or HMO against too great a loss and is provided by larger insurance companies. Reinsurance is used most frequently by small insurers. If insurance expenses exceed an agreed upon amount then reinsurance would pay for this unexpectedly large amount that might otherwise bankrupt the insurer.

Private (Nongovernment) Health Insurance

The two major types of private providers of insurance are Blue Cross–Blue Shield and insurance companies.

Blue Cross–Blue Shield. "The Blues" are independent (nongovernment, private), nonprofit, tax-exempt corporations providing primarily protection against the costs of hospital care (Blue Cross), and surgery and other types of physician care (Blue Shield) in a limited geographic area (usually a state).

If there was a single starting point for Blue Cross, it was the prepayment plan for Dallas teachers established at Baylor University by Justin F. Kimball in 1929. This program enrolled 1,250 school teachers who paid 50¢ a month to be eligible for up to twenty-one days of semiprivate hospitalization at Baylor University Hospital. The American Hospital Association endorsed this prepayment idea in 1933. The next year the Blue Cross symbol was first used to designate nonprofit hospital plans. By 1938, the basic principles for Blue Cross plans were established.

- They are nonprofit organizations.
- The board of directors are to represent hospitals, physicians, and the public.
- They are to be supervised by state insurance departments.
- They hold low cash reserves.
- They emphasize hospital benefits in the form of service, rather than cash indemnities.
- The plans are not to be in competition with each other, and therefore do not have overlapping geographical boundaries.
- Employees are on salary and salesmen are not paid on commission.

By 1937, the state medical societies of California, Michigan, and Pennsylvania were sponsoring physician service plans. In 1946, the AMA financed the Associated Medical Care Plans, which became the National Association of Blue Shield Plans. In 1960, the Blue Cross Association became the sole national federation of Blue Cross plans.

Until 1978 Blue Cross and Blue Shield (the Blues, or BC–BS, or BX) were legally independent of each other, but often worked in close cooperation, offering matched benefit packages to insured groups. They have since merged at the national level and in many states.

There are approximately seventy Blue Cross organizations covering part of a state (Associated Hospital Service of New York), an entire state (Massachusetts Blue Cross), or several states (Vermont and New Hampshire). They are linked as members of the Blue Cross Association, which provides shared services and arranges for coverage with other Blue Cross plans for travelers who leave their own plan's area. Blue Cross is set up in most states under special enabling legislation, generally providing that it should be regulated by the state insurance department. In some states Blue Cross must submit to public hearings before it can raise its rates.

Until 1972 the American Hospital Association owned the Blue Cross symbol and set requirements for corporations using this symbol, including that it (1) cover a large enough area, (2) provide service benefits, (3) have a contract with the majority of hospitals in its area, and (4) have at least one-third of the board representing the public and one-third representing the contracting hospitals.

Blue Cross calls these features that distinguish it from other private insurance companies "prepayment" rather than "insurance." It provides *service benefits* (as opposed to direct cash payments to insured persons to pay for care, which are called *indemnity benefits*) that consist of a contract benefit which is paid directly to the provider of hospital or medical care for services rendered. This requires a contractual agreement between the insurer and provider of care (hospitals and Blue Cross, doctors and Blue Shield), and distinguishes the Blue Cross–Blue Shield plans from the commercial insurers who make payments to the (beneficiary) patient, not the provider. The Blue Cross contract usually specifies what the hospital is allowed to charge the patients covered by Blue Cross. The hospitals are not limited in this way with patients covered by commercial insurance policies.

Blue Cross Enabling Legislation.   Although the contents of this legislation varies from state to state, it usually includes the following:

- Blue Cross and Blue Shield are allowed to operate in the state.
- The state insurance commissioner is given certain powers to regulate the plan.

- Premium rate increases must be approved by the insurance commissioner after a public hearing.

- Blue Cross and Blue Shield are the only organizations that are allowed to contract with providers for service benefits at agreed upon charges.

Private Insurance Companies.[6]   About 1,100 private insurance companies write health insurance using thousands of policies. Some major companies include Prudential, Equitable, Aetna, Metropolitan, and Connecticut General. In 1850 individual accident insurance first became available in the United States and by 1866 more than 60 insurors provided accident insurance. In 1910 Montgomery Ward and Company started what was probably the first group health insurance program for their employees. In the 1940s, during World War II, wages were frozen and therefore employee health insurance benefits became a major part of collective bargaining between unions and employers. (Commercial insurance companies then entered the field in increasing numbers.)

In 1977, 9 out of 10 people under 65 (167,000,000) had some form of nongovernment health insurance, although the range and adequacy of coverage varies widely. Of these, 92.8 million persons were covered by private companies—91.9 by group contracts. (Blue Cross–Blue Shield covered 79 million and 18.9 million had other coverage, including health maintenance organizations.) In addition, 6 out of 10 persons over 65 had policies supplementing Medicare; these are often called "medigap" policies and these too vary greatly in range and adequacy.

A growing number of large employers (those with several thousand employees) have created their own health insurance funds for their employees. When an employee uses insured medical care the employer pays for it out of this fund, often using an independent insurance agency to pay the bills and keep track of records and expenditures.

---

6. These are sometimes called *commercial insurance companies*. The word "commercial" is not used by the companies in this category and has ideological implications related to the competition between these companies and Blue Cross–Blue Shield.

Health Maintenance Organizations

A *health maintenance organization* (HMO) may be broadly defined as an organization that is responsible for the provision of relatively comprehensive health services to enrolled persons in return for a set monthly fee (premium). The HMO provides services directly or by contract with specific providers. The term was introduced by Paul Ellwood in 1971[7] to refer to a group of independent insurance plans, including Kaiser–Permanente in California, which had combined prepayment (capitation) with group practice. The term was popularized by the federal government, which encouraged this form of health insurance because of its apparent record of effective cost control associated with lower rates of hospital use.

The capitation payment method to the provider of service that is at the core of the HMO concept is not new. In 1721 in Boston, Dr. William Douglas offered his patients the option of paying fee-for-service or by a fixed yearly amount; "five pounds per annum sick or well."[8] Perhaps the first of the recent HMOs was the Western Clinic of Tacoma, Washington. This group of doctors formed in 1906 and agreed to a prepaid capitation contract with a lumber company in about 1910.[9]

Table 5–1 lists a few well-known HMOs, their locations, starting dates, and major sponsors. Table 5–2 lists seven major dimensions of HMOs that can be combined in different ways.

There are two basic types of HMOs. *Prepaid group practices* (PGPs) such as Kaiser–Permanente; and *individual practice associations* (IPAs), some of which are also called *foundations for medical care* (see p. 269) and comprise physicians in independent practice. PGPs include organized groups of physicians and a capitation mechanism. IPAs were developed by local medical societies. Participating individual physicians charge fee-for-service and submit to peer utilization review. Physician and hospital reimbursement come from the

7. Paul M. Ellwood et al., "Health Maintenance Strategy," *Medical Care* 9 (1971): 291.

8. From a letter to Cadwallader Colden. "Letters from Dr. William Douglas to Cadwallader Colden of New York," *Collections of the Massachusetts Historical Society*, 4th series, vol. 2, 1854, pp. 164–189.

9. Robert Shouldice and Katherine H. Shouldice, *Medical Group Practice and Health Maintenance Organizations* (Washington, D.C.: Information Resources Press, 1978).

Table 5-1. Some Well-Known HMOs.

Name	Location	Date Started	Sponsor
Ross Loos Clinic	Los Angeles	1929	Medical partnership
Community Hospital Association	Elk City Oklahoma	1929	Cooperative
Group Health Cooperative of Puget Sound	Seattle	1935	Cooperative
Kaiser Foundation Health Plan	Several states, Headquarters in Oakland, California	1942	Industry
Health Insurance Plan of Greater New York	New York City	1946	City, physicians, and community
Harvard Community Health Plan	Boston	1969	University

In 1980 there were approximately 235 health maintenance organizations which had enrolled about 9,100,000 persons. About half of these were federally qualified.

subscribers' capitation payments. Individual participating physicians can also care for patients outside of the IPA plan. The initially clear distinction between IPAs and PGPs have blurred together in some cases. For example, IPAs can contract with pre-existing group practices. Complex payment formulas for doctors and hospitals have developed and differ from one plan to another.

In many people's minds the Kaiser-Permanente Health Plan typifies the HMO. Although it is not the oldest HMO, it is by far the largest. It includes the following characteristics:

Financing and provision of care are combined.

Fixed premium payment "prepayment": Community-rated fixed monthly dues paid primarily through the members' place of employment.

Medical group practice: Made up of full-time physicians paid on a capitation, rather than a fee-for-service basis.

Hospital based: The group practice is generally physically combined with an owned and operated hospital.

Table 5-2. Dimensions of Health Maintenance Organizations (HMOs).

Relation with Hospital	Relations with Physicians	Form of Medical Practice	Formation of Groups	Spacial Arrangement	Type of Organization	Qualification
(1) Owns hospital	(4) Employs groups of physicians	(7) Physicians in groups	(9) Group practice formed by HMO	(11) Physicians and hospital generally in same location	(13) Not for profit	(15) Federally qualified
(2) Contracts with hospital	(5) Contracts primarily with individual physicians	(8) Individual physicians	(10) Group in existence prior to HMO affiliation	(12) Physicians and hospital generally in separate locations	(14) For profit	(16) Not federally qualified
(3) No special relationship with hospital	(6) Contracts primarily with group practices					

Examples: Kaiser Foundation Health Plan — (1), (6), (7), (9), (11), (13), (15)
Harvard Community Health Plan — (1), (2), (4), (7), (8), (12), (13), (15)
Foundation Health Plan (Sacramento, California) — (2), (5), (7), (8), (10), (12), (13), (15)
Intergroup Prepaid Health Services, Inc. (Chicago) — (3), (6), (7), (10), (12), (14), (15)

Voluntary enrollment: People are given the option of joining this plan or having some other coverage such as Blue Cross–Blue Shield.

Capitation payments: Payments to hospital (Kaiser) and doctors (Permanente) are on a fixed monthly basis regardless of use.

Comprehensiveness: A wide range of benefits are provided without deductibles or coinsurance.

Nonprofit, nongovernment organization.

Nearly every one of these basic characteristics has, in one way or another, been modified by other HMOs.

Some HMOs separate financing and provision of care. For example, Blue Cross–Blue Shield may receive payments from enrollees and pass them on to the corporately independent HMO. The "Blues" are actively promoting over sixty HMOs throughout the country. Medicaid and Medicare allow for enrollment in HMOs with payment from government funds. Some HMOs contract with small groups of physicians or solo practitioners, paying them on a capitation basis. Some HMOs do not own their own hospital or their group practice is physically separate from the hospital.

Voluntary enrollment continues to exist everywhere, although now employees may confront five or more choices. Comprehensiveness varies with the plan. There are HMOs run on a for-profit basis, and others formed by medical societies, labor unions, universities, insurance companies, cooperatives, and other organizations on a nonprofit basis.

Multiple choice of health plans at the place of employment is seen by some as a competitive way of introducing more cost control into medical care. This is developing into one of the unique features of American medical care. Usually each year the employee may choose from several different health plans that may include one or more HMOs, a Blue Cross plan, or a commercial insurance plan. (For example, U.S. government employees in Washington, D.C. have five choices.) The plans have different benefits and sometimes different prices per month (monthly premium payments). In some companies the employees who choose a lower cost plan have less money removed from their paycheck (payroll deduction), thereby giving them a money incentive to choose an efficient plan. Most of the costs of medical care insurance are paid by the employer for the employee and the amount paid and range of benefits are often the subject of labor-management negotiations along with other fringe benefits such as life insurance, pension plans, and educational benefits.

Because the employer pays for medical care this is a business expense and not taxable for the employer, nor is it subject to employee federal income tax. If employees paid for the coverage themselves, they would first have to pay federal, state, and possibly local income tax on the earned income. This provides an economic advantage to have the employer pay for more medical care benefits and the employee less.

Federal Definition of an HMO

The U.S. government defines HMOs in the following terms.[10] They provide basic health services to enrollees and supplemental benefits for additional payment. Prepayment enrollment fees are fixed uniformly on a community-rated basis (requirements recently modified) regardless of the patient's medical history. Basic health services include physicians' services; inpatient, outpatient, and emergency care; crisis mental health care; care for drug abuse and alcohol addiction; x-ray and laboratory tests; home health care; and preventive services. Supplemental care may include long-term care, vision care, dental services, other mental health services, long-term physical medicine, and prescription drugs.

Services are provided by HMO staff or professionals under contract. Medically necessary services must be available twenty-four hours a day, seven days a week. There must be reimbursement for emergency care, provided outside the HMO service area. The physicians must have a prearranged way of distributing the HMO income.

The HMO must be financially sound. There must be open annual enrollment with no more than 75 percent enrollment from a medically underserved population. One-third of the board of directors must be enrollees. Health education services must be provided. There must be an ongoing quality assurance program. The HMO must report statistical and cost information to the federal government.

---

10. For purposes of eligibility for grant funds under the Health Maintenance Organization Act, P.L. 93-222.

HMOs that can or attempt to fulfill these conditions, *federally qualified HMOs*, are eligible for certain benefits under PL 93–222. This federal law supersedes restrictive state laws, some of which limited HMO growth. Employers of twenty-five or more workers who receive health benefits are required to offer an HMO option if there is a qualified HMO in the area.

Workmen's Compensation

Workmen's compensation[11] (industrial accident insurance) is an example of governmental social insurance. It started in the first decade of this century. In 1948 all states had workmen's compensation, in addition to the Federal Employees Compensation Act (FECA, passed in 1908, replaced in 1916, and amended in 1949 by PL 81–357). These laws are based on the idea that the employer is financially liable for injuries to employees, although the employee does not have to prove that the employer was negligent.

There are three categories of benefits: (1) cash; (2) medical; and (3) rehabilitation to indemnify the worker injured on the job or his or her dependents for loss of wages, medical and hospital expenses, and loss of occupational capacity and skills. These benefits are financed by employers, either through insuring with a private insurance company or, in some states, through a state fund or by self-insurance. Benefits vary substantially from state to state and by type of employment.

THE FLOW OF FUNDS IN THE HEALTH CARE SYSTEM

Payments for governmental health insurance (Medicare) are made in relationship to place of employment. The employee and employer pay social security taxes (employer contribution and employee's payroll deduction). Insurance, Blue Cross, or other coverage for the employee and his or her family (dependents) is also customarily obtained at the place of employment (employee benefit plans). The

---

11. For a good review of workmen's compensation see that section in *Social Security Programs in the United States*, a publication of the Social Security Administration, Department of Health and Human Services, which is issued periodically.

employee pays through payroll deductions and the employer usually contributes to the premium as a fringe benefit. (Fringe benefits are nonsalary compensations, such as health and life insurance and retirement benefits.) Blue Cross provides payments directly to the provider (vendor) in the form of service benefits. These providers are under contract. Insurance companies have no contractual arrangement with providers (usually this is forbidden by state insurance laws). Insurance companies pay benefits directly to the subscriber who, in turn, pays the provider. The subscriber may *assign* his or her benefits to the provider and then the insurance company will send its benefit directly to the provider. In addition, there are *out-of-pocket* (or direct) expenses paid directly by the user to the provider. (Persons who choose to have no health insurance or to pay a large deductible are said to be *self-insured*.)

Federal, state, and local governments provide funds through their various health care systems and, especially on the federal level, through an extensive system of government grants to the public and nonprofit sectors (see Chapter 6). The government also pays providers of care through the Medicaid program.

The government (for Medicare and Medicaid), Blue Cross–Blue Shield, and insurance companies are referred to as *third party payers* (the other "parties" being patient and provider). The agreement between providers (usually hospitals) and third party payers (usually Blue Cross and government programs) as to what, and how much, will be paid for is called the *reimbursement formula*. These can be extremely complicated. For example, "cost or charges, whichever is less" means that the third party payer will pay either the provider's actual costs, or what it ordinarily charges patients, whichever figure is lower.

Prospective reimbursement means that the payer and the provider agree in advance on a budget for the provider and, therefore, on the provider's expected costs. If the provider's services cost more, then the provider must absorb the loss. If the provider's services cost less, the provider keeps the extra. Prospective reimbursement and other formulas that try to encourage efficient provider performance are called *incentive reimbursement. Preadmission (prospective) screening of admissions* means that the doctor or hospital must receive prior approval from the payer to admit an elective patient, in order to be reimbursed. *Retrospective denial of payment* means that the payer reviews the appropriateness of the use of services, after they have been used. If the payer finds the services provided were medically unnecessary, it will not reimburse the provider for them.

Payment for most physicians and virtually all dentists is on a *fee-for-service* basis. A fee is charged for each service with differing fees according to the length and difficulty of the procedure.

A *relative value scale* is a listing of services and procedures performed. Each is given an index number that reflects the relative length and difficulty of the task. This index can then be multiplied by a fixed dollar amount to obtain an appropriate fee. The California Relative Value Scale is the best known of these scales. Such scales are now viewed by the Federal Trade Commission as possible devices to fix prices and limit competition and as a result, their use has diminished.

The fee for a given procedure that is usually charged by the physician and other physicians in the area is called a *usual and customary fee*.

Physicians in group practice are paid according to a variety of arrangements determined by the group. In the case of prepaid group practice, the group as a whole is paid by *capitation* (according to the number of persons or families enrolled). The income is then distributed to the physician in an agreed upon way. Physicians who work in government health systems and other organizations, such as some HMOs, outpatient departments, and health centers, are paid by salary.

Charitable Contributions

Prior to the advent of Medicare and Medicaid, philanthropic gifts were a major source of funds for medical care, especially for the poor. Traditionally, hospital trustees were expected to contribute substantially to the financing of their hospitals. Physicians were expected to contribute part of their time to care of the poor without pay. Often they were required to cover hospital clinics in exchange for admitting privileges at the hospital. House staff obtained much of their training caring for the poor for little or no pay. Many religious organizations, particularly the Roman Catholic Church, have played important roles in funding care for the poor.

Since the advent of Medicare and Medicaid this type of philanthropy has greatly diminished, especially in hospitals, although endowment funds developed from past philanthropy remain significant for many organizations. Now philanthropy is more focused on studies, demonstration programs, research, and education. Many voluntary organizations, however, such as the Red Cross and the American Cancer Society, rely heavily on donations; volunteers give many hours to medical service organizations, and voluntary donations of blood are of great importance.

NATIONAL HEALTH EXPENDITURE DATA

- National health expenditures have been rising and account for a growing share of the *gross national product* (the value of all goods and services produced in the country during the year)—from 4.5 percent in 1950 to 9.0 percent in 1979. See Figure 5–2 and Table 5–3.[12]

- The proportion of health care expenditures paid by the government has been increasing from 27 percent in 1950 to 43.0 percent in 1979. See Table 5–3.

- The proportion of health care expenses consumed by hospitals has risen from 30 percent in 1950 to 40.2 percent in 1979. See Table 5–4.

- Federal government health expenditures are greater than state and local government expenditures, $56.4 billion versus $28.8 billion, respectively, in 1979. See Table 5–6.

- In terms of total dollars spent by government, Medicare ($30.3 billion) and Medicaid ($22.7 billion) are the two single largest programs. See Table 5–6.

12. This was 9.4 percent in 1980.

Figure 5-2. National Health Expenditures and Percent of Gross National Product, Selected Calendar Years, 1950–1979.

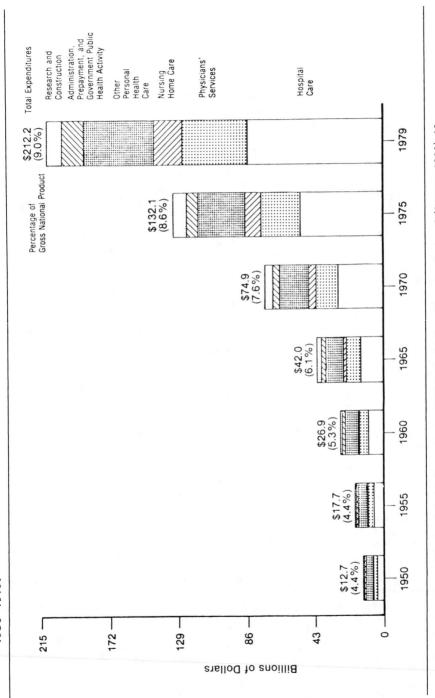

Source: Robert Gibson, "National Health Expenditures, 1979," *Health Care Financing Review* 2 (Summer 1980): 12.

Table 5-3. National Health Expenditures: Amount and Per Capita Amount by Major Source of Funds and Percentage of Gross National Product, Selected Calendar Years, 1929-1979.

	1979	1978	1977	1976	1975	1974
National Health Expenditures (billions)	$212.2	$188.6	$169.9	$148.9	$132.1	$116.3
As a Percent of the GNP	9.0%	8.9%	8.9%	8.7%	8.6%	8.2%
Sources of Funds:						
Private Expenditures	$120.8	$108.0	$99.3	$85.7	$75.8	$69.1
Public Expenditures	91.4	80.7	70.6	63.2	56.3	47.2
Federal Expenditures	60.9	53.9	47.4	42.6	37.1	30.5
State/Local Expenditures	30.5	26.8	23.2	20.6	19.2	16.7
Per Capita Expenditures[a]	$942.94	$845.53	$768.30	$678.79	$607.58	$539.1
Sources of Funds:						
Private Expenditures	$536.82	$483.88	$448.93	$390.59	$348.63	$320.4
Public Expenditures	406.12	361.64	319.38	288.21	258.95	218.6
Federal Expenditures	270.80	241.58	214.47	194.21	170.52	141.2
State/Local Expenditures	135.32	120.06	104.91	93.99	88.43	77.3
Percentage Distribution of Funds	100.00%	100.00%	100.00%	100.00%	100.00%	100.0
Private Funds	56.93	57.23	58.43	57.54	57.38	59.4
Public Funds	43.07	42.77	41.57	42.46	42.62	40.5
Federal Funds	28.72	28.57	27.91	28.61	28.07	26.2
State/Local Funds	14.35	14.20	13.66	13.85	14.55	14.3
Addenda:						
Gross National Product (billions)	$2,368.8	$2,127.6	$1,899.5	$1,702.2	$1,528.8	$1,412.9
Population (thousands)	225,041	223,107	221,104	219,318	217,452	215,696
Annual Percentage Changes						
National Health Expenditures	12.5	11.0	14.1	12.7	13.6	12.8
Private Expenditures	11.9	8.8	15.9	13.0	9.7	8.5
Public Expenditures	13.3	14.3	11.7	12.3	19.4	19.8
Federal Expenditures	13.1	13.7	11.3	14.9	21.7	21.2
State/Local Expenditures	13.7	15.5	12.5	7.2	15.2	17.4
Gross National Product	11.3	12.0	11.6	11.3	8.2	8.1
Population	.9	.9	.8	.9	.8	.8

a. Based on July 1 population estimates including outlying territories, armed forces, and Federal employees overseas and their dependents.

Source: Robert Gibson, "National Health Expenditures, 1979," *Health Care Financing Review* 2 (Summer 1980): 16.

Table 5-3. continued

1973	1972	1971	1970	1965	1960	1950	1940	1929
$103.0	$93.5	$83.1	$74.9	$42.0	$26.9	$12.7	$4.0	$3.6
7.9%	8.0%	7.8%	7.6%	6.1%	5.3%	4.4%	4.0%	3.5%
$63.7	$58.1	$51.4	$47.1	$31.0	$20.3	$9.2	$3.2	$3.2
39.4	35.4	31.7	27.8	11.0	6.6	3.4	.8	.5
25.1	22.8	20.3	•17.6	5.6	3.0	1.6	n.a.	n.a.
14.2	12.6	11.4	10.2	5.3	3.6	1.8	n.a.	n.a.
$481.65	$440.34	$394.74	$359.41	$212.32	$146.30	$81.86	$29.62	$29.49
$297.72	$273.44	$244.28	$225.98	$156.84	$110.20	$59.62	$23.61	$25.49
183.94	166.90	150.47	133.44	55.48	36.10	22.24	6.03	4.00
117.52	107.50	96.32	84.53	28.44	16.42	10.49	n.a.	n.a.
66.41	59.40	54.15	48.90	27.04	19.69	11.75	n.a.	n.a.
100.00%	100.00%	100.00%	100.00%	100.00%	100.00%	100.00%	100.00%	100.00%
61.81	62.10	61.88	62.87	73.87	75.32	72.83	79.66	86.43
38.19	37.90	38.12	37.13	26.13	24.68	27.17	20.34	13.57
24.40	24.41	24.40	23.52	13.39	11.22	12.81	n.a.	n.a.
13.79	13.49	13.72	13.61	12.74	13.46	14.36	n.a.	n.a.
$1,306.5	$1,171.1	$1,063.4	$982.4	$688.1	$506.0	$286.2	$100.0	$103.4
213,941	212,338	210,546	208,402	197,784	183,831	154,675	134,591	123,731
10.2	12.5	11.0	12.3	9.3	7.8	12.2	.8	
9.7	12.9	9.2	8.7	8.9	8.2	11.2	.1	
11.0	11.9	13.9	20.4	10.6	6.8	15.5	4.6	
10.1	12.6	15.1	25.7	13.3	6.4	n.a.	n.a.	
12.6	10.6	11.9	13.8	8.1	7.1	n.a.	n.a.	
11.6	10.1	8.2	7.4	6.3	5.9	11.1	-.3	
.8	.9	1.0	1.1	1.5	1.7	1.4	.8	

Table 5-4. National Health Expenditures by Type of Expenditure, Amount, Per Capita Amount, and Percentage Distribution, Selected Years, 1929–1979.

Type of Expenditure	1979	1976	1970	1960	1950	1940	1929
				Amount (in millions)			
Total	$212,199	$148,872	$74,903	$26,895	$12,662	$3,987	$3,649
Health Services and Supplies	202,318	139,823	69,583	25,185	11,702	3,868	3,436
Personal Health Care	188,551	131,276	65,372	23,680	10,885	3,548	3,202
Hospital Care	85,342	59,808	27,799	9,092	3,851	1,011	663
Physicians' Services	40,599	27,565	14,340	5,684	2,747	973	1,004
Dentists' Services	13,607	9,448	4,750	1,977	961	419	482
Other Professional Services	4,687	3,202	1,595	862	396	174	252
Drugs and Medical Sundries	16,975	12,781	8,208	3,657	1,726	637	606
Eyeglasses and Appliances	4,353	3,219	1,926	776	491	189	133
Nursing Home Care	17,807	11,390	4,697	526	187	33	—
Other Health Services	5,180	3,863	2,058	1,106	526	112	62
Prepayment and Administration	7,720	4,734	2,791	1,091	456	167	139
Government Public Health Activities	6,047	3,813	1,420	414	361	153	96
Research and Construction of Medical Facilities	9,882	9,049	5,320	1,710	960	119	213
Research[b]	4,615	3,635	1,889	662	117	3	—
Construction	5,267	5,414	3,431	1,048	843	116	213
				Per Capita Amount[a]			
Total	$942.94	$678.79	$359.41	$146.30	$81.86	$29.62	$29.49
Health Services and Supplies	899.03	637.53	333.89	137.00	75.66	28.74	27.77
Personal Health Care	837.85	598.57	313.68	128.81	70.37	26.36	25.88
Hospital Care	379.23	272.70	133.39	49.46	24.90	7.51	5.36
Physicians' Services	180.41	125.69	68.81	30.92	17.76	7.23	8.11
Dentists' Services	60.46	43.08	22.79	10.75	6.21	3.11	3.90
Other Professional Services	20.83	14.60	7.65	4.69	2.56	1.29	2.04

Drugs and Medical Sundries	75.43	58.28	39.39	19.89	11.16	4.73	4.90
Eyeglasses and Appliances	19.34	14.68	9.24	4.22	3.17	1.40	1.07
Nursing Home Care	79.13	51.93	22.54	2.86	1.21	.25	—
Other Health Services	23.02	17.62	9.87	6.02	3.40	.83	.50
Prepayment and Administration	34.31	21.58	13.39	5.93	2.95	1.24	1.12
Government Public Health Activities	26.87	17.38	6.81	2.25	2.33	1.14	.78
Research and Construction of							
Medical Facilities	43.91	41.26	25.53	9.30	6.21	.88	1.72
Research b	20.51	16.57	9.06	3.60	.76	.02	—
Construction	23.40	24.69	16.46	5.70	5.45	.86	1.72

Percentage Distribution

Total	100.00%	100.00%	100.00%	100.00%	100.00%	100.00%	100.00%
Health Services and Supplies	95.3	93.9	92.9	93.6	92.4	97.0	94.2
Personal Health Care	88.9	88.2	87.3	88.0	86.0	89.0	87.8
Hospital Care	40.2	40.2	37.1	33.8	30.4	25.4	18.2
Physicians' Services	19.1	18.5	19.1	21.1	21.7	24.4	27.5
Dentists' Services	6.4	6.3	6.3	7.4	7.6	10.5	13.2
Other Professional Services	2.2	2.2	2.1	3.2	3.1	4.4	6.9
Drugs and Medical Sundries	8.0	8.6	11.0	13.6	13.6	16.0	16.6
Eyeglasses and Appliances	2.1	2.2	2.6	2.9	3.9	4.7	3.6
Nursing Home Care	8.4	7.7	6.3	2.0	1.5	.8	—
Other Health Services	2.4	2.6	2.7	4.1	4.2	2.8	1.7
Prepayment and Administration	3.6	3.2	3.7	4.1	3.6	4.2	3.8
Government Public Health Activities	2.9	2.6	1.9	1.5	2.9	3.8	2.6
Research and Construction of							
Medical Facilities	4.7	6.1	7.1	6.4	7.6	3.0	5.8
Research b	2.2	2.4	2.5	2.5	.9	.1	—
Construction	2.5	3.6	4.6	3.9	6.7	2.9	5.8

a. Based on July 1 population estimates including outlying territories, armed forces and Federal employees overseas, and their dependents.

b. Research and development expenditures of drug companies and other manufacturers and providers of medical equipment and supplies are excluded from "research expenditures," but included in the expenditure class in which the product falls.

Source: Robert Gibson, "National Health Expenditures, 1979," *Health Care Financing Review* 2 (Summer 1980):21 and 22.

Table 5-5. Personal Health Care Expenditures by Selected Third-Party Payers and Type of Expenditure, Amount, Per Capita Amount, and Percentage Distribution, 1979.

Source of Payment	Total	Hospital Care	Physicians' Services	Dentists' Services	Other Professional Services	Drugs and Medical Sundries	Eyeglasses and Appliances	Nursing Home Care	Other Health Services
					Amount (in millions)				
Total	188,551	85,342	40,599	13,607	4,687	16,975	4,353	17,807	5,180
Direct Payments	59,973	6,905	14,813	9,938	2,832	14,216	3,789	7,481	—
Third-Party Payments	128,578	78,437	25,786	3,669	1,855	2,760	564	10,326	5,180
Private Health Insurance	50,286	29,803	15,138	3,130	604	1,339	155	117	—
Philanthropy and Industrial In-Plant	2,407	942	24	—	52	—	—	107	1,283
Government	75,884	47,692	10,624	539	1,200	1,420	409	10,102	3,897
Federal	53,311	34,886	7,999	298	848	705	332	5,461	2,783
Medicare [a]	29,328	21,651	6,407	—	552	—	249	373	97
Medicaid [b]	11,770	4,347	1,203	243	249	665	—	4,775	287
Other	12,213	8,888	389	54	47	39	82	313	2,399
State and Local	22,573	12,806	2,625	241	352	716	77	4,642	1,114
Medicaid [b]	9,913	3,662	1,015	205	210	560	—	4,021	241
Other	12,660	9,144	1,611	36	143	155	77	621	874
					Per Capita Amount [c]				
Total	$837.85	$379.23	$180.41	$60.46	$20.83	$75.43	$19.34	$79.13	$23.02
Direct Payments	266.50	30.68	65.82	44.16	12.58	63.17	16.84	33.24	—
Third-Party Payments	571.35	348.54	114.59	16.30	8.25	12.26	2.51	45.89	23.02
Private Health Insurance	223.45	132.43	67.27	13.91	2.68	5.95	.69	.52	—
Philanthropy and Industrial In-Plant	10.70	4.18	.11	—	.23	—	—	.48	5.70

	100.0%	100.0%	100.0%	100.0%	100.0%	100.0%	100.0%	100.0%	100.0%
Government	337.20	211.93	47.21	2.39	5.33	6.31	1.82	44.89	17.32
Federal	236.90	155.02	35.55	1.32	3.77	3.13	1.47	24.27	12.37
Medicare a	130.32	96.21	28.47	—	2.45	—	1.11	1.66	.43
Medicaid b	52.30	19.32	5.35	1.08	1.11	2.96	—	21.22	1.28
Other	54.27	39.50	1.73	.24	.21	.18	.37	1.39	10.66
State and Local	100.31	56.90	11.66	1.07	1.57	3.18	.34	20.63	4.95
Medicaid b	44.05	16.27	4.51	.91	.93	2.49	—	17.87	1.07
Other	56.26	40.63	7.16	.16	.63	.69	.34	2.76	3.88

Percentage Distribution

Total	100.0%	100.0%	100.0%	100.0%	100.0%	100.0%	100.0%	100.0%	100.0%
Direct Payments	31.8	8.1	36.5	73.0	60.4	83.7	87.0	42.0	—
Third-Party Payments	68.2	91.9	63.5	27.0	39.6	16.3	13.0	58.0	100.0
Private Health Insurance	26.7	34.9	37.3	23.0	12.9	7.9	3.6	.7	—
Philanthropy and Industrial In-Plant	1.3	1.1	.1	—	1.1	—	—	.6	24.8
Government	40.2	55.9	26.2	4.0	25.6	8.4	9.4	56.7	75.2
Federal	28.3	40.9	19.7	2.2	18.1	4.2	7.6	30.7	53.7
Medicare a	15.6	25.4	15.8	—	11.8	—	5.7	2.1	1.9
Medicaid b	6.2	5.1	3.0	1.8	5.3	3.9	1.9	26.8	5.5
Other	6.5	10.4	1.0	.4	1.0	.2	1.8	1.8	46.3
State and Local	12.0	15.0	6.5	1.8	7.5	4.2	1.8	26.1	21.5
Medicaid b	5.3	4.3	2.5	1.5	4.5	3.3	—	22.6	4.6
Other	6.7	10.7	4.0	.3	3.0	.9	1.8	3.5	16.9

a. Represents total expenditures from trust funds for benefits. Trust fund income includes premium payments paid by or on behalf of beneficiaries.

b. Includes funds paid into Medicare trust funds by States under "buy-in" agreements to cover premiums for public assistance recipients and for persons who are medically indigent.

c. Based on July 1 population estimates including outlying territories, armed forces and Federal employees overseas, and their dependents.

(Table 5-5. continued overleaf)

Table 5-5 (continued). Personal Health Care Expenditures by Selected Third-Party Payers and Type of Expenditure, Amount, Per Capita Amount, and Percentage Distribution, 1975.

Source of Payment	Total	Hospital Care	Physicians' Services	Dentists' Services	Other Professional Services	Drugs and Medical Sundries	Eyeglasses and Appliances	Nursing Home Care	Other Health Services
					Amount (in millions)				
Total	116,522	52,141	24,932	8,237	2,619	11,813	2,982	10,105	3,692
Direct Payments	37,725	3,978	8,682	6,412	1,596	10,048	2,725	4,284	–
Third-Party Payments	78,797	48,164	16,250	1,825	1,022	1,766	257	5,821	3,692
Private Health Insurance	31,077	18,766	9,684	1,358	420	738	32	78	892
Philanthropy and Industrial In-Plant	1,539	542	14	–	29	–	–	61	892
Government	46,182	28,855	6,552	467	573	1,027	226	5,681	2,800
Federal	31,531	20,253	4,665	275	375	527	174	3,186	2,076
Medicare[a]	15,588	11,603	3,338	–	199	–	114	291	43
Medicaid[b]	7,431	2,642	1,048	205	139	498		2,720	179
Other	8,512	6,009	278	70	37	30	61	174	1,854
State and Local	14,650	8,602	1,887	192	198	500	51	2,496	723
Medicaid[c]	5,873	2,087	828	162	110	393	–	2,150	141
Other	8,778	6,515	1,059	30	88	107	51	346	582
					Per Capita Amount[c]				
Total	$535.85	$239.78	$114.66	$37.88	$12.04	$54.33	$13.72	$46.47	$16.98
Direct Payments	173.49	18.29	39.93	29.49	7.34	46.21	12.53	19.70	–
Third-Party Payments	362.37	221.49	74.73	8.39	4.70	8.12	1.18	26.77	16.98
Private Health Insurance	142.91	86.30	44.53	6.24	1.93	3.40	.15	.36	–
Philanthropy and Industrial In-Plant	7.08	2.49	.06	–	.13	–	–	.28	4.10

	100.0%	100.0%	100.0%	100.0%	100.0%	100.0%	100.0%	100.0%	100.0%
Government	212.38	132.70	30.13	2.15	2.64	4.72	1.04	26.13	12.87
Federal	145.00	93.14	21.45	1.26	1.72	2.42	.80	14.65	9.55
Medicare a	71.69	53.36	15.35	–	.91	–	.52	1.34	.20
Medicaid b	34.17	12.15	4.82	.94	.64	2.29	–	12.51	.82
Other	39.15	27.63	1.28	.32	.17	.14	.28	.80	8.53
State and Local	67.37	39.56	8.68	.88	.91	2.30	.23	11.48	3.33
Medicaid b	27.01	9.60	3.81	.75	.51	1.81	–	9.89	.65
Other	40.37	29.96	4.87	.14	.41	.49	.23	1.59	2.68

Percentage Distribution

Total	100.0%	100.0%	100.0%	100.0%	100.0%	100.0%	100.0%	100.0%	100.0%
Direct Payments	32.4	7.6	34.8	77.8	61.0	85.1	91.4	42.4	–
Third-Party Payments	67.6	92.4	65.2	22.2	39.0	14.9	8.6	57.6	100.0
Private Health Insurance	26.7	36.0	38.8	16.5	16.0	6.3	1.1	.8	24.2
Philanthropy and Industrial In-Plant	1.3	1.0	.1	–	1.1	–	–	.6	–
Government	39.6	55.3	26.3	5.7	21.9	8.7	7.6	56.2	75.8
Federal	27.1	38.8	18.7	3.3	14.3	4.5	5.8	31.5	56.2
Medicare a	13.4	22.3	13.4	–	7.6	–	3.8	2.9	1.2
Medicaid b	6.4	5.1	4.2	2.5	5.3	4.2	–	26.9	4.8
Other	7.3	11.5	1.1	.8	1.4	.3	2.0	1.7	50.2
State and Local	12.6	16.5	7.6	2.3	7.6	4.2	1.7	24.7	19.6
Medicaid b	5.0	4.0	3.3	2.0	4.2	3.3	–	21.3	3.8
Other	7.5	12.5	4.2	.4	3.4	.9	1.7	3.4	15.8

a. Represents total expenditures from trust funds for benefits. Trust fund income includes premium payments paid by or on behalf of beneficiaries.

b. Includes funds paid into Medicare trust funds by States under "buy-in" agreements to cover premiums for public assistance recipients and for persons who are medically indigent.

c. Based on July 1 population estimates including outlying territories, armed forces and Federal employees overseas, and their dependents.

(Table 5-5. continued overleaf)

Table 5-5 (continued). Personal Health Care Expenditures by Selected Third-Party Payers and Type of Expenditure, Amount, Per Capita Amount, and Percentage Distribution, 1970.

Source of Payment	Total	Hospital Care	Physicians' Services	Dentists' Services	Other Professional Services	Drugs and Medical Sundries	Eyeglasses and Appliances	Nursing Home Care	Other Health Services
					Amount (in millions)				
Total	65,372	27,799	14,340	4,750	1,595	8,208	1,926	4,697	2,058
Direct Payments	26,128	2,816	6,328	4,286	1,094	7,414	1,815	2,375	—
Third-Party Payments	39,244	24,983	8,012	463	500	794	111	2,322	2,058
Private Health Insurance	15,744	10,008	4,908	240	262	310	3	12	—
Philanthropy and Industrial In-Plant	1,040	384	10	—	20	—	—	34	592
Government	22,460	14,591	3,093	223	218	484	108	2,276	1,466
Federal	14,561	9,428	2,232	130	138	239	79	1,339	976
Medicare[a]	7,098	4,978	1,720	—	77	—	46	259	18
Medicaid[b]	2,795	1,225	380	91	41	226	—	779	53
Other	4,669	3,226	133	39	20	13	33	301	905
State and Local	7,899	5,163	861	93	80	245	29	938	490
Medicaid[b]	2,310	1,012	314	75	34	187	—	644	44
Other	5,589	4,151	547	18	46	59	29	294	445
					Per Capita Amount[c]				
Total	$313.68	$133.39	$68.81	$22.79	$7.65	$39.39	$9.24	$22.54	$9.87
Direct Payments	125.37	13.51	30.37	20.57	5.25	35.57	8.71	11.39	—
Third-Party Payments	188.31	119.88	38.44	2.22	2.40	3.81	.53	11.14	9.87
Private Health Insurance	75.54	48.02	23.55	1.15	1.26	1.49	.01	.06	—
Philanthropy and Industrial In-Plant	4.99	1.84	.05	—	.10	—	—	.16	2.84

Government	107.77	70.01	14.84	1.07	1.05	2.32	.52	10.92	7.03
Federal	69.87	45.24	10.71	.62	.66	1.15	.38	6.42	4.69
Medicare [a]	34.06	23.89	8.25	—	.37	—	.22	1.24	.08
Medicaid [b]	13.41	5.88	1.82	.44	.20	1.08	—	3.74	.26
Other	22.40	15.48	.64	.19	.09	.06	.16	1.44	4.34
State and Local	37.90	24.77	4.13	.45	.39	1.18	.14	4.50	2.35
Medicaid [b]	11.08	4.86	1.51	.36	.16	.90	—	3.09	.21
Other	26.82	19.92	2.63	.08	.22	.28	.14	1.41	2.14

Percentage Distribution

Total	100.0%	100.0%	100.0%	100.0%	100.0%	100.0%	100.0%	100.0%	100.0%
Direct Payments	40.0	10.1	44.1	90.2	68.6	90.3	94.2	50.6	—
Third-Party Payments	60.0	89.9	55.9	9.8	31.4	9.7	5.8	49.4	100.0
Private Health Insurance	24.1	36.0	34.2	5.1	16.5	3.8	.1	.3	—
Philanthropy and Industrial In-Plant	1.6	1.4	.1	—	1.3	—	—	.7	28.8
Government	34.4	52.5	21.6	4.7	13.7	5.9	5.6	48.5	71.2
Federal	22.3	33.9	15.6	2.7	8.6	2.9	4.1	28.5	47.4
Medicare [a]	10.9	17.9	12.0	—	4.8	—	2.4	5.5	.9
Medicaid [b]	4.3	4.4	2.6	1.9	2.6	2.8	—	16.6	2.6
Other	7.1	11.6	.9	.8	1.2	.2	1.7	6.4	44.0
State and Local	12.1	18.6	6.0	2.0	5.0	3.0	1.5	20.0	23.8
Medicaid [b]	3.5	3.6	2.2	1.6	2.1	2.3	—	13.7	2.1
Other	8.5	14.9	3.8	.4	2.9	.7	1.5	6.3	21.6

a. Represents total expenditures from trust funds for benefits. Trust fund income includes premium payments paid by or on behalf of beneficiaries.

b. Includes funds paid into Medicare trust funds by States under "buy-in" agreements to cover premiums for public assistance recipients and for persons who are medically indigent.

c. Based on July 1 population estimates including outlying territories, armed forces and Federal employees overseas, and their dependents.

(Table 5-5. continued overleaf)

Table 5-5 (continued). Personal Health Care Expenditures by Selected Third-Party Payers and Type of Expenditure, Amount, Per Capita Amount, and Percentage Distribution, 1965.

Source of Payment	Total	Hospital Care	Physicians' Services	Dentists' Services	Other Professional Services	Drugs and Medical Sundries	Eye-glasses and Appliances	Nursing Home Care	Other Health Services
					Amount (in millions)				
Total	$36,000	$13,885	$8,473	$2,809	$1,033	$5,212	$1,211	$2,072	$1,306
Direct Payments	18,584	2,374	5,197	2,717	897	4,881	1,181	1,337	—
Third-Party Payments	17,416	11,510	3,276	92	136	331	30	735	1,306
Private Health Insurance	8,729	5,790	2,680	43	79	135	1	2	—
Philanthropy and Industrial In-Plant	788	309	8	—	18	—	—	21	431
Government	7,899	5,412	588	49	39	197	29	712	875
Federal	3,785	2,430	151	32	12	120	12	460	568
Medicare[a]	—	—	—	—	—	—	—	—	—
Medicaid[b]	—	—	—	—	—	—	—	—	—
Other	3,785	2,430	151	32	12	120	12	460	568
State and Local	4,114	2,982	436	17	26	76	17	251	308
Medicaid[b]	—	—	—	—	—	—	—	—	—
Other	4,114	2,982	436	17	26	76	17	251	308
					Per Capita Amount[c]				
Total	$182.02	$70.20	$42.84	$14.20	$5.22	$26.35	$6.12	$10.48	$6.60
Direct Payments	93.96	12.00	26.28	13.74	4.54	24.68	5.97	6.76	—
Third-Party Payments	88.06	58.20	16.56	.46	.69	1.67	.15	3.72	6.60
Private Health Insurance	44.13	29.27	13.55	.22	.40	.68	.01	.01	—
Philanthropy and Industrial In-Plant	3.98	1.56	.04	—	.09	—	—	.11	2.18

Government	39.94	27.36	2.97	.25	.20	.99	.15	3.60	4.43
Federal	19.14	12.28	.76	.16	.06	.61	.06	2.33	2.87
Medicare[a]	–	–	–	–	–	–	–	–	–
Medicaid[b]	–	–	–	–	–	–	–	–	–
Other	19.14	12.28	.76	.16	.06	.61	.06	2.33	2.87
State and Local	20.80	15.08	2.21	.08	.13	.39	.08	1.27	1.55
Medicaid[b]	–	–	–	–	–	–	–	–	–
Other	20.80	15.08.	2.21	.08	.13	.39	.08	1.27	1.55
Percentage Distribution								
Total	100.0%	100.0%	100.0%	100.0%	100.0%	100.0%	100.0%	100.0%	100.0%
Direct Payments	51.6	17.1	61.3	96.7	86.9	93.6	97.5	64.5	–
Third-Party Payments	48.4	82.9	38.7	3.3	13.1	6.4	2.5	35.5	100.0
Private Health Insurance	24.2	41.7	31.6	1.5	7.6	2.6	.1	.1	–
Philanthropy and Industrial In-Plant	2.2	2.2	.1	–	1.8	–	–	1.0	–
Government	21.9	39.0	6.9	1.7	3.7	3.8	2.4	34.3	33.0
Federal	10.5	17.5	1.8	1.1	1.2	2.3	1.0	22.2	67.0
Medicare[a]	–	–	–	–	–	–	–	–	–
Medicaid[b]	–	–	–	–	–	–	–	–	–
Other	10.5	17.5	1.8	1.1	1.2	2.3	1.0	22.2	43.5
State and Local	11.4	21.5	5.1	.6	2.5	1.5	1.4	12.1	23.5
Medicaid[b]	–	–	–	–	–	–	–	–	–
Other	11.4	21.5	5.1	.6	2.5	1.5	1.4	12.1	23.5

a. Represents total expenditures from trust funds for benefits. Trust fund income includes premium payments paid by or on behalf of beneficiaries.

b. Includes funds paid into Medicare trust funds by States under "buy-in" agreements to cover premiums for public assistance recipients and for persons who are medically indigent.

c. Based on July 1 population estimates including outlying territories, armed forces and Federal employees overseas, and their dependents.

Source: Robert Gibson, "National Health Expenditures, 1979," *Health Care Financing Review* 2 (Summer 1980): 29–32.

Table 5-6. Expenditures for Health Services and Supplies Under Public Programs by Program, Type of Expenditure, and Source of Funds (*in millions*) 1979.

| Program Area | Total | Health Services and Supplies | | | |
| | | Personal Health Care | | | |
		Total	Hospital Care	Physicians Services	Dentists Services
All Public Programs	85,237	75,884	47,692	10,624	539
Total Federal Expenditures	56,439	53,311	34,886	7,999	298
Total State and Local Expenditures	28,798	22,573	12,806	2,625	241
Major Program Areas:					
Medicare[a]	30,338	29,328	21,651	6,407	—
Medicaid[b]	22,796	21,683	8,009	2,217	448
Federal Expenditures	12,464	11,770	4,347	1,203	243
State and Local Expenditures	10,332	9,913	3,662	1,015	205
Other Public Assistance Payments for Medical Care	1,530	1,530	565	157	32
Federal Expenditures	—	—	—	—	—
State and Local Expenditures	1,530	1,530	565	157	32
Veterans' Medical Care	5,355	5,305	4,444	61	36
Department of Defense Medical Care[c]	4,023	4,000	2,837	107	2
Workers Compensation	4,442	3,342	1,696	1,411	—
Federal Employees	108	108	71	27	—
State and Local Programs	4,333	3,233	1,625	1,384	—
State and Local Hospitals (net)[d]	6,828	6,828	6,828	—	—
Other Public Expenditures for Personal Health Care[e]	3,879	3,869	1,662	265	22
Federal	2,810	2,800	1,536	195	17
State and Local	1,069	1,069	125	70	5
Government Public Health Activities	6,047	—	—	—	—
Federal	1,341	—	—	—	—
State and Local	4,706	—	—	—	—

a. Represents total expenditures from trust funds for benefits and administrative costs Trust fund income includes premium payments paid by or on behalf of beneficiaries.

b. Includes funds paid into Medicare trust funds by States under "buy-in" agreements to cover premiums for public assistance recipients and for persons who are medically indigent.

c. Includes care for retirees and military dependents. Payments for services other than hospital care and other health services represent only those made under contract medical programs.

Table 5-6. continued

| | Health Services and Supplies | | | | | |
| | Personal Health Care | | | | | Govern-ment Public Health Activities |
Other Profes-sional Services	Drugs and Medical Sundries	Eye-glasses and Appliances	Nursing Home Care	Other Health Services	Admin-istration	
1,200	1,420	409	10,102	3,897	3,306	6,047
848	705	332	5,461	2,783	1,787	1,341
352	716	77	4,642	1,114	1,519	4,706
552	—	249	373	97	1,010	—
459	1,226	—	8,796	528	1,113	—
249	665	—	4,775	287	694	—
210	560	—	4,021	241	419	—
32	86	—	621	37	—	—
—	—	—	—	—	—	—
32	86	—	621	37	—	—
—	13	48	313	391	50	—
—	11	—	—	1,043	23	—
103	66	66	—	—	1,100	—
6	2	2	—	—	—	—
96	64	64	—	—	1,100	—
—	—	—	—	—	—	—
55	18	46	—	1,801	10	—
40	14	33	—	965	10	—
14	5	13	—	836	—	—
—	—	—	—	—	—	6,047
—	—	—	—	—	—	1,341
—	—	—	—	—	—	4,706

d. Expenditures for State and local government hospitals not offset by other revenues.

e. Includes program spending for Maternal and Child Health; Vocational Rehabilitation medical payments; Temporary Disability Insurance medical payments; PHS and other Federal hospitals; Indian Health Services; Alcoholism, Drug Abuse, and Mental Health; and school health.

SELECTED READINGS

Blue Cross Since 1929, Odin Anderson (Cambridge, Mass.: Ballinger Publishing Company, 1975).

Health Maintenance Organizations: A Guide to Planning and Development, Roger W. Birnbaum (New York: Spectrum Publications, 1976).

Source Book of Health Insurance Data, Health Insurance Institute, New York (Yearly).

"Financing for Health Care," Carol McCarthy. In Steven Jonas and contributors, *Health Care Delivery in the United States*, 2nd edition (New York: Springer Publishing Co., 1981).

Medical Group Practice and Health Maintenance Organizations, Robert Shouldice and Katherine Shouldice (Washington, D.C.: Information Resources Press, 1978).

The Kaiser Permanente Medical Care Program, A Symposium, Anne R. Somers (New York: The Commonwealth Fund, 1971).

6 THE FEDERAL GOVERNMENT AND HEALTH

There is no constitutionally defined role for the federal government in health and therefore such activities have been traditionally reserved to the states. Nevertheless, over the years there has been a gradual development of a federal presence in the field of health, a presence that has greatly increased in the past twenty-five years. The sources of this still expanding role include:

- The special responsibility for certain population groups, such as merchant seamen, members of the armed forces, veterans, and American Indians;

- The Constitutional power to regulate interstate commerce; much of the regulatory power of the federal government in health as in other areas derives from this power. An example is the regulation of food and drugs.

- Grants-in-aid to states, institutions, and individuals for a wide variety of activities; and

- Most recently, sponsorship and financial participation in the health insurance program for the elderly (Medicare).

EXECUTIVE AGENCIES

Laws passed by Congress, the legislative branch of the federal government, are implemented and administered by the many departments, agencies, and bureaus of the executive branch. Implementation is effected by rules and regulations that are written and promulgated in the *Federal Register* by these agencies and have the force of law. These rules are codified in the *Code of Federal Regulations.*

Many of these administrative bodies have primarily a service function, such as overseeing the distribution of federal funds; regulation and control is in the context of seeing that funds are used and services provided in accordance with the intent of the relevant statutes. Examples are the Medicare and Medicaid bureaus of the Health Care Financing Administration; and the Centers for Disease Control (CDC), which, among other activities, provide, at the request of state health departments, assistance in the investigation of disease outbreaks.[1]

Other agencies are primarily regulatory in function. Some of these are independent, such as the Federal Trade Commission and the Product Safety Commission. Others are part of cabinet departments, such as the Food and Drug Administration and the Occupational Safety and Health Administration, but even these have considerable autonomy within the executive branch.[2]

Many of the procedures of the executive agencies are quasi-judicial; hearings and appeals are adjudicated by *administrative law judges* (formerly known as hearing officers or hearing examiners and deployed by the Civil Service Commission). Agency decisions may be appealed to the federal courts, but not until all review and appeals procedures have been exhausted.

The power to make regulations and adjudicate is in effect delegated to the administrative bodies by Congress and general proce-

---

1. For example, staff from the CDC participated with personnel from the Pennsylvania and Philadelphia Health Departments in the investigation of the 1976 outbreak of Legionnaires' Disease. Scientists from the Center were ultimately successful in isolating the responsible organism.

2. The first of the federal regulatory agencies was the Interstate Commerce Commission, established in 1887 to regulate the railroads. The most recent are the Environmental Protection Agency (1970), the Occupational Safety and Health Administration (1970), and the Consumer Product Safety Commission (1972).

dures for the agencies were explicitly set forth in the Administrative Procedures Act of 1946.

Deregulation. In recent years there has been increasing pressure in Congress, by Presidential administrations, and by regulated groups for simplification and de-emphasis of the federal regulatory process. This has resulted in regulatory changes ranging from the reduction of the numbers of regulations[3] and the clarification of their language, to the actual repeal of laws regulating entire industries (e.g., the airline industry). The deregulation process is continuing at an accelerated rate and includes, in addition to reduction in regulatory activity, such controversial proposals and measures as congressional review of regulations ("legislative veto"), restrictions on the functions of regulatory agencies, and the application of cost–benefit evaluations to regulation writing.

Most federal health-related functions are consolidated in the various units of the Department of Health and Human Services (formerly the Department of Health, Education and Welfare). Many functions, however, are among the responsibilities of a variety of other departments, agencies, and bureaus, where they generally represent only a part of or are incidental to the main activities of the unit. The more important of these are briefly noted below.

Executive Office of the President

Office of Management and Budget. This office was organized in 1970, replacing the Bureau of the Budget. It is responsible for the preparation, supervision, and control of the federal budget and for the overall administration and management of the executive branch. Thus, this agency greatly affects the operation and activities of all federal agencies.

---

3. In 1977 for example, the Occupational Safety and Health Administration withdrew some 1,000 regulations deemed of little usefulness for the protection of workers. There have also been many reductions of regulations by other agencies.

Cabinet Departments

Department of Agriculture. This department is responsible through its *Food Safety and Quality Service* for the inspection of meat, poultry, and egg products processed by plants shipping in interstate or foreign commerce, and for the voluntary inspection and grading of foods. The *Food and Nutrition Service* administers the food stamp program and the school lunch and school breakfast programs. The Supplemental Food Program for Women, Infants and Children (WIC Program) provides food supplements and nutrition counseling for low-income pregnant and nursing women and children up to age five through facilities such as health centers and outpatient departments.

Department of Defense. This department is responsible for the health and medical care of members of the armed forces through the Assistant Secretary for Health and Environment. A complete range of health and medical care programs, institutions, and training programs is operated (see p. 8). Civilian medical care for dependents of active duty, retired, or deceased servicemen is administered through the CHAMPUS insurance program (Civilian Health and Medical Program of the Uniformed Services). An armed forces medical school (Uniformed Services University of the Health Sciences) in Bethesda, Maryland was established under 1972 legislation (Uniformed Services Revitalization Act). The first class graduated in 1980.

Department of Housing and Urban Development. This department's programs of assistance for urban development and improvement, especially in low income areas, include, under *community development block grant* programs, options for improvement of neighborhood health services.[4]

Department of Education. Formerly the Office of Education in the Department of Health, Education and Welfare, this agency was given cabinet status by Congress in 1980, and certain educational programs from other federal agencies were added to it. Its health related re-

---

4. Health related activities were features of many "Model Cities" programs, which preceded the Housing and Community Development Act of 1974.

sponsibilities include support of programs directed to the education and rehabilitation of the handicapped[5] and to health, alcohol, and drug abuse education.

The department also sets standards and criteria for the recognition, for purpose of federal funding, of voluntary agencies that accredit educational institutions and programs, including those engaged in health manpower education and training.

The American Printing House for the Blind, Gallaudet College (for the deaf), and the National Technical Institute for the Deaf at the Rochester Institute of Technology are supported in part by funds appropriated in the department's budget.

Department of Justice. The *Drug Enforcement Administration* (DEA) is responsible for federal control of narcotics and other drugs subject to abuse (under the Controlled Substances Act of 1970). It regulates the manufacture, distribution, and dispensing of such drugs. Physicians, pharmacists, and other professionals who prescribe or dispense drugs must register with the DEA.

Department of Labor. This department's *Occupational Safety and Health Administration* is responsible for the promotion of industrial health and safety and the enforcement of related laws and regulations.[6] The *Mine Safety and Health Administration* is responsible for control of health and safety hazards in the mining industry.

Independent Agencies

There are many federal agencies that are not part of cabinet departments or the executive office. They include a wide variety of administrations, agencies, boards, commissions, councils, and so forth. Among those with some health related activities are the following.

ACTION. This agency was established in 1971 to incorporate a number of national volunteer programs, including the Peace Corps (for international volunteers) and the domestic volunteer program

---

5. Under the Rehabilitation Act of 1973 and Education for All Handicapped Children Act of 1975.

6. The department's activities in this area were considerably expanded by the Occupational Safety and Health Act of 1970.

VISTA (Volunteers in Service to America), the Foster Grandparent Program, and the Retired Senior Volunteer Program.

Advisory Commission on Intergovernmental Relations. This is a twenty-six-member body established by Congress in 1959 to provide a continuing review of the federal system as it relates to state and local governments. Its membership represents federal, state, and local government and the general public. The commission publishes annual reports that are of considerable general interest.

Appalachian Regional Commission. This commission was created in 1965 by the Appalachian Redevelopment Act. It consists of a representative of each of thirteen eastern states,[7] a federal co-chairman, and a state governor (in rotation) as co-chairman. The purpose of the commission is to promote the economic, physical, and social development of the region. The commission sponsors a variety of health projects, including community health clinics and manpower training programs.

Consumer Product Safety Commission. This commission was created by the Consumer Product Safety Act (1972) to develop safety standards and regulations related to consumer products. The Commission also assumed responsibility for administering existing legislation including the Flammable Fabrics Act and the Poisoning Prevention Packaging Act. It has the authority to ban from interstate commerce certain categories of products it deems hazardous.

Environmental Protection Agency. This agency was established in 1970 to coordinate and consolidate federal activities in environmental quality control. Its responsibilities include implementation of the Clean Air Act, the Federal Water Pollution Control Act, the Solid Waste Disposal Act, and the Safe Drinking Water Act.

Federal Trade Commission. This commission has responsibilities in the area of federal trade regulation of trade in interstate commerce, including prevention of unfair or deceptive practices and unfair methods of competition. Recent activities in the health field have

7. The Appalachian region, for purposes of the Commission, includes portions of thirteen states: Alabama, Georgia, Kentucky, Maryland, Mississippi, New York, North Carolina, Ohio, Pennsylvania, South Carolina, Tennessee, Virginia, and West Virginia.

included inquiries into practices it deems anticompetitive by health professionals and institutions (including advertising prohibitions, relative value scales, and certain accreditation procedures). It also regulates the labeling and advertising of nonprescription over-the-counter (OTC) drugs.

Occupational Safety and Health Review Commission. This is an adjudicating agency established by the Occupational Safety and Health Act of 1970 to rule on cases of disagreement over the enforcement actions of the Occupational Safety and Health Administration.

Veterans Administration. The Veterans Administration's (VA's) *Department of Medicine and Surgery* administers the program of medical services for veterans of the armed forces who have service-related illnesses and disabilities, or are medically indigent. Services are rendered through an extensive network of VA hospitals, clinics, nursing homes, and residential units, as well as non–VA facilities and practitioners. These services are supported by a variety of related manpower training activities including an extensive internship and residency program (see also p. 11).

Quasi-Official Agencies

There are a number of agencies that, while not formally a part of the federal government, have a special statutory relationship to it. These include the National Academy of Sciences and the American Red Cross.

National Academy of Sciences. Established by an Act of Congress in 1863, the Academy consists of scientists elected in recognition of their research contributions. It acts as the official advisor to the federal government in matters of science and technology. It also includes the National Academy of Engineering and two operating arms, the National Research Council (1916) and the Institute of Medicine (1970).

American Red Cross. Founded by Clara Barton in 1881 and chartered by an Act of Congress in 1905 the American Red Cross (formerly American National Red Cross) serves members of the armed forces and is an official agency for domestic and international war and disaster relief.

THE DEPARTMENT OF HEALTH, EDUCATION AND WELFARE (1953-1980)

The Department of Health, Education and Welfare (HEW), now the Department of Health and Human Services, was created in 1953 by elevating to cabinet status the Federal Security Agency, which included most of the federal health, education, and social welfare agencies functioning at that time. These included the Public Health Service, the Food and Drug Administration, the Social Security Administration (which included the Children's Bureau), the Office of Education, and the Office of Vocational Rehabilitation (see Figure 6-1).

Public Health Service. The U.S. Public Health Service was the oldest of HEW's component agencies. It was established by Congress in 1798 as the Marine Hospital Service for the "relief of sick and disabled seamen." This care was financed by monthly contributions of twenty cents from each merchant seaman's wages. The Service was placed in the Treasury Department (where it remained until 1939), and the tax was collected by the Collector of Customs.[8] Gradually, a number of special marine hospitals were constructed in principal ports.

In 1878 the Service was authorized by Congress to develop recommendations for uniform quarantine laws and regulation in the states and to carry out investigations related to the cause and control of epidemic disease. Thereafter, its functions steadily increased. Notable dates are the following:

1887 – A research program was begun with the establishment of the Hygienic Laboratory at the Marine Hospital on Staten Island, New York.

---

8. Later this tax, the first U.S. compulsory sickness insurance, was discontinued and costs were paid from general revenues.

Figure 6-1. Department of Health, Education, and Welfare, 1953.*

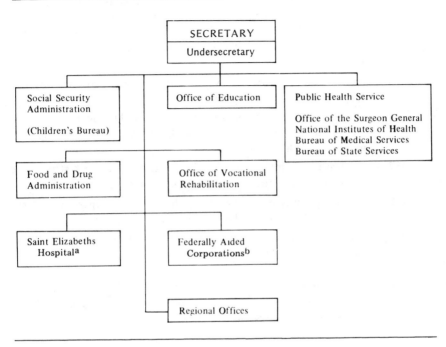

*Abbreviated.

a. A psychiatric hospital for residents of the District of Columbia and persons eligible for care by the Public Health Service or Veterans' Administration.

b. The federally aided corporations are supported in part by federal funds appropriated in the budget of the Department of Health, Education and Welfare. They are: *American Printing House for the Blind, Columbia Institute for the Deaf* (Kendall School and Gallaudet College), *Howard University.*

1889 — The professional personnel were organized in a quasimilitary Commissioned Corps under a Surgeon General who became the chief executive officer of the Public Health Service.[9]

1893 — The Service was given full responsibility for foreign and interstate quarantine.

1902 — The Service was reorganized and renamed the Public Health and Marine Hospital Service. It was given responsibility for licensing and regulating the interstate sale of biological products. The Surgeon

9. Initially, members of the Corps were physicians. Membership was broadened by Acts of Congress in 1930 and 1944 to include other professionals.

General was authorized to call an annual conference of state and territorial health officers.

1912 — The service was renamed the U.S. Public Health Service. In subsequent years, its added responsibilities included the National Leprosarium (Carville, Louisiana), a hospital for the treatment of narcotic addicts (Lexington, Kentucky), and a Venereal Disease Control division.

1930 — The Hygienic Laboratory was redesignated the National Institute of Health.

1935 — The Social Security Act's Title VI, administered by the Public Health Service, authorized grants-in-aid to the states for strengthening state and local health departments.

1937 — The National Cancer Act created the National Cancer Institute, the first specialty institute in the National Institute of Health.

1939 — The Service was transferred from the Treasury Department to the newly established Federal Security Agency.

1944 — The Public Health Service Act of 1944 revised substantially and brought together in one statute all existing legislation concerning the Public Health Service.

1946 — The Communicable Disease Center was established in Atlanta, Georgia. The Census Bureau's Division of Vital Statistics was transferred to the service as the National Office of Vital Statistics.

Food and Drug Administration. This agency, known until 1931 as the *Food, Drug, and Insecticide Administration*, was established in the Department of Agriculture in 1927. It replaced the *Bureau of Chemistry* in administering the several existing acts relating to the quality and safety of food and drugs, including the Pure Food and Drug Act. It was transferred to the Federal Security Agency in 1940. (Responsibility for the inspection of meat and poultry remained with the Department of Agriculture.)

Social Security Administration. The Social Security Administration (originally the Social Security Board) administered the sections of the Social Security Act related to Old Age and Survivors Insurance ("social security"), federal aid to state programs for public assistance ("welfare"), and unemployment insurance. This agency also included the important Children's Bureau.

Children's Bureau. The Children's Bureau was created within the Department of Labor in 1912 to "investigate and report upon . . .

all matters pertaining to the welfare of children and child life. . . ."
During the next decade it developed an extensive program of studies,
research, and distribution of educational material relating to the
health and welfare of mothers and children.

1921 — The Maternity and Infancy Act (Sheppard–Towner Act) provided
grants to the states for promotion of maternal and child health care
and greatly expanded the scope and activities of the Bureau. Maternal and child health units were subsequently established in many
states previously without them.

1929 — The Maternity and Infancy Act expired and the activities of the
Bureau were subsequently curtailed.

1935 — Title V of the Social Security Act provided grants-in-aid to the
states for maternal and child health, child welfare, and crippled children. The responsibilities of the bureau were again greatly increased.

1946 — The Children's Bureau was transferred from the Department of
Labor to the Social Security Administration in the Federal Security
Agency.

1943 — The Bureau administered until 1949 the Emergency Maternity and
Infant Care Program for dependents of servicemen.

Office of Education.   The Office of Education was established in the
Department of the Interior in 1867 to gather statistics and facts and
to diffuse information concerning education. Added responsibilities
included the administration of grants-in-aid to land grant colleges
(1890), and grants to the states for vocational rehabilitation programs (1920 to 1943) and vocational education programs (1933).
The office became part of the Federal Security Agency in 1939.

Office of Vocational Rehabilitation.   The Office of Vocational Rehabilitation was established in 1943 to administer an expanded program of grants to the states for vocational rehabilitation of disabled
persons (under the Vocational Rehabilitation Act Amendments of
1943).

Reorganizations

The Department of Health, Education and Welfare (HEW) was reorganized many times during the twenty-seven years of its existence as
such. In 1963, the *Welfare Administration* was established to admin-

ister the public assistance and related social service programs. The Children's Bureau was also transferred to this agency, as were the Office of Aging and the Office of Juvenile Delinquency and Youth Development (from the Office of the Secretary of HEW). In 1967, the Welfare Administration and the Vocational Rehabilitation Administration were absorbed into the new *Social and Rehabilitation Service*.

In 1968, the Public Health Service was reorganized with the creation of the *Health Services and Mental Health Administration* (HSMHA) to incorporate most of the traditional functions of the service. The Service was placed under the direction of the Assistant Secretary for Health and Scientific Affairs with the Surgeon General his principal deputy.

Another noteworthy reorganization involved the Children's Bureau. In 1969, the Bureau was moved from the Social and Rehabilitation Service to the new *Office of Child Development*. Its health programs were placed in the new Maternal and Child Health Service (part of HSMHA) and its social service programs were merged with programs for adults in the Social and Rehabilitation Service. The Bureau retained responsibility for overall coordination of maternal and child health programs, and its original mandate to investigate and report upon matters relating to health and welfare of children. The Office of Child Development also now included the *Head Start* program transferred from the Office of Economic Opportunity.

The general organization of HEW in 1972 is shown in Figure 6-2. The Health Services and Mental Health Administration is shown in Table 6-1.

In July 1973, the health agencies of the Department of Health, Education and Welfare were again extensively reorganized. HSMHA was replaced by two new units, the *Health Services Administration* and the *Health Resources Administration*. The Center for Disease Control became a separate agency, and the National Institute of Mental Health became part of a new *Alcohol, Drug Abuse and Mental Health Administration*. Finally, the functions of the Bureau of Health Manpower Education were transferred from the National Institutes of Health to the new Health Resources Administration.

Additional changes were also made in the Office of the Secretary of HEW. Among these was the establishment of the position of Assistant Secretary of Human Development, whose responsibilities included the Office of Child Development, Office of Youth Develop-

Figure 6-2. Department of Health, Education, and Welfare, 1972.*

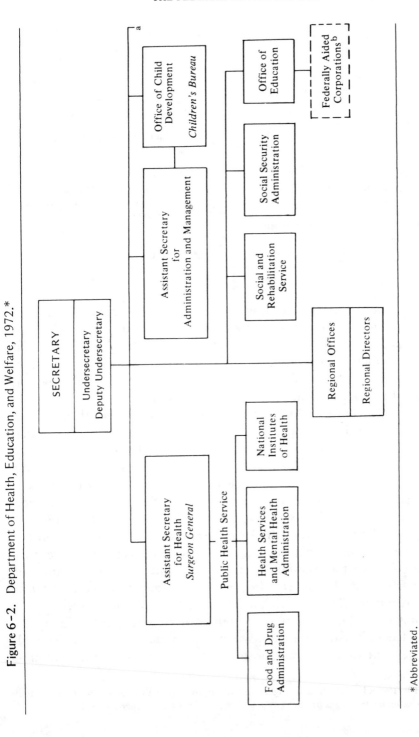

*Abbreviated.

a. Also Assistant Secretaries for: Public Affairs, Community and Field Services, Legislation, and Planning and Evaluation.

b. American Printing House for the Blind, Gallaudet College, Howard University.

Table 6-1.   Health Services and Mental Health Administration, 1972.

Development	Health Services Delivery
National Center for Health Services Research and Development	National Center for Family Planning Services
Health Care Facilities Service	Maternal and Child Health Service
Comprehensive Health Planning Service	Community Health Service
Regional Medical Programs Service	Indian Health Service
Health Maintenance Organization Service	Federal Health Programs Service
	National Health Service Corps
Prevention and Consumer Services	**Mental Health**
Center for Disease Control	National Institute of Mental Health
National Institute of Occupational Safety and Health	National Institute on Alcohol Abuse and Alcoholism
Bureau of Community Environmental Management	

National Center for Health Statistics

ment, and the Administration on Aging.[10] In 1975 the Rehabilitation Services Administration (formerly the Vocational Rehabilitation Administration) was also transferred to this office from the Social and Rehabilitation Service. An *Office of Inspector General* was established in the Office of the Secretary in 1976. The general organization of the Department in 1976 is shown in Figure 6-3.

In 1977, another extensive reorganization of the health and social welfare agencies of the department was carried out. A new *Health Care Financing Administration* was established, to assume primary responsibility for the Medicare and Medicaid programs. It took over the functions of the Bureau of Health Insurance (Medicare) from the Social Security Administration, the Medical Services Administration (Medicaid) from the Social and Rehabilitation Service, the Bureau of Quality Assurance from the Health Services Administration and the Offices of Professional Standards Review and Long Term Care from the Office of the Assistant Secretary of Health. A reorganization of the Office of Human Development (now named *Office of Human Development Services*) included the transfer of social services programs from the Social and Rehabilitation Service. Responsibility for the federally aided public assistance program Aid to Families with Dependent Children was transferred to the Social Security Adminis-

10. The Administration on Aging was transferred from the Social and Rehabilitation Service under provisions of the 1973 amendments of the Older Americans Act.

Figure 6-3. Department of Health, Education and Welfare, 1976.*

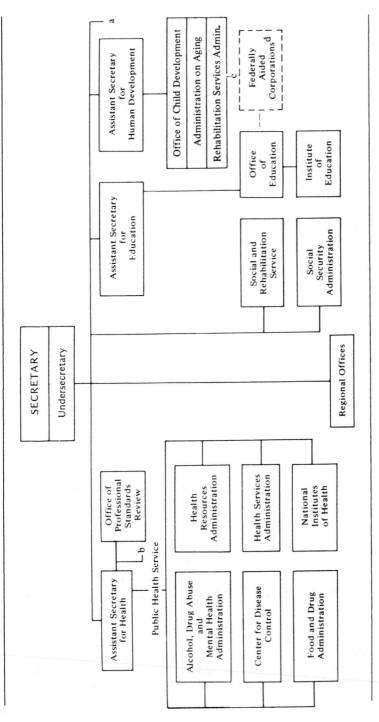

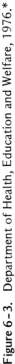

*Abbreviated.

a. Also Assistant Secretaries for Public Affairs, Legislation, Planning and Evaluation, Administration and Management, and a Comptroller.

b. Also: Office of International Health, Office of Population Affairs, Office of Nursing Home Affairs.

c. Also: Office of Youth Development, Office for Handicapped Individuals, Office of Native American Programs, Office of Rural Development.

d. American Printing House for the Blind, Gallaudet College, Howard University.

tration from the Social and Rehabilitation Service. The latter agency was abolished.

In 1978 the National Center for Health Services Research and the National Center for Health Statistics were moved from the Health Resources Administration to the Office of the Assistant Secretary for Health, where a new *National Center for Health Care Technology* was also established.

In 1980, with the establishment of the new cabinet level Department of Education, the Department of Health, Education and Welfare became the *Department of Health and Human Services*.

THE DEPARTMENT OF HEALTH
AND HUMAN SERVICES

The Department of Health and Human Services (HHS), formerly the Department of Health, Education and Welfare, is the major health agency of the federal government, and has a budget second only to that of the Department of Defense. It consists of four major operating agencies: the Public Health Service, the Health Care Financing Administration, the Social Security Administration, and the Office of Human Development Services. The general organization of HHS in 1981 is shown in Figure 6–4.

Public Health Service

The Public Health Service is under the direction of the Assistant Secretary for Health. The Surgeon General is his principal deputy. The Surgeon General was for many years the chief executive officer of the Public Health Service and the senior public health officer of the Commissioned Corps.[11] With the reorganization of 1968, which gave line authority to the Assistant Secretary, the role of Surgeon General was de-emphasized. The post has at times been left vacant; more recently, it was combined with that of the Assistant Secretary. It is now again a separate position.

---

11. The Commissioned Corps, analogous in organization to the other uniformed services, consists of about 7,000 professionals: physicians, dentists, nurses, dieticians, engineers, pharmacists, physical therapists, sanitarians, scientists, veterinarians, and other professionals. Professionals are also employed by the Service under the Civil Service General Schedule (GS) personnel system.

Figure 6–4. Department of Health and Human Services, 1981.*

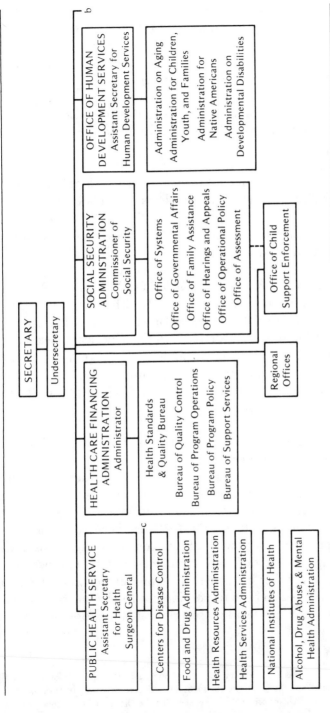
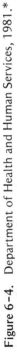

*Abbreviated.

a. The Inspector General and Assistant Secretaries for Public Affairs, Legislation, Planning, and Evaluation, Management and Budget; and Personnel Administration.

b. Office of Adolescent Pregnancy Programs, Office of Health Information, Health Promotion and Physical Fitness and Sports Medicine, Office of Health Maintenance Organizations, and Office on Smoking and Health.

The Service now comprises six agencies: the Alcohol, Drug Abuse and Mental Health Administration (ADAMHA), the Centers for Disease Control (CDC), the Food and Drug Administration (FDA), the Health Resources Administration (HRA), the Health Services Administration (HSA), and the National Institutes of Health (NIH).

Alcohol, Drug Abuse and Mental Health Administration.   This agency was established in 1973 and incorporated the following three institutes:

National Institute on Alcohol Abuse and Alcoholism.   Responsible for programs directed toward the problems of alcohol abuse.

National Institute on Drug Abuse.   Administers programs directed to the problems of drug abuse.

National Institute of Mental Health.   Established in 1946 as the second specialty institute of the Public Health Service. It was separated from the National Institutes of Health as a separate bureau in 1967 and in 1968 was incorporated into the new Health Services and Mental Health Administration. It administers programs of research, service development, and training in mental health. *St. Elizabeths Hospital* [12] has been nominally under the auspices of the Institute since 1967.

Centers for Disease Control (CDC).   The Centers developed from the Communicable Disease Center, which was renamed Center for Disease Control in 1970 when its functions were broadened to address, in addition to its traditional activities related to infectious disease, other preventable conditions, including malnutrition. A major and longstanding responsibility of the CDC has been the conduct and support of programs for prevention and control of infectious disease, and providing consultation and assistance to state and local health departments and other countries, including extensive epidemiological services. It has also been responsible for foreign quarantine activities. Since 1967 it has also licensed clinical laboratories in interstate commerce.

---

12. St. Elizabeths Hospital was established by Congress in 1855 (as a "Government Hospital for the Insane") in the setting of the mental health reform efforts of Dorothea Dix. It now provides psychiatric care primarily for residents of the District of Columbia.

Under the 1973 Public Health Service reorganization, the CDC incorporated the National Institute of Occupational Safety and Health (NIOSH),[13] including the Appalachian Laboratory of Occupational Respiratory Disease; and took over from the former Bureau of Community Environmental Management the functions related to lead poisoning prevention and rat control. *The Bureau of Health Education*, including the National Clearing House on Smoking and Health, was added in 1975.

In 1980 the Center for Disease Control was reorganized and renamed *Centers for Disease Control*. The Centers are:

- Center for Infectious Diseases
- Center for Prevention Services
- Center for Environmental Health
- Center for Health Promotion and Education
- Center for Professional Development and Training
- National Institute for Occupational Safety and Health.

In addition there are the Epidemiology Program Office, International Program Office, and Laboratory Improvement Office. The headquarters of the CDC is in Atlanta, Georgia.

Food and Drug Administration. This agency is responsible for the safety of foods,[14] drugs, medical devices, biologics, cosmetics, and radiation-emitting equipment; for proper labeling and product information; and approval of all new drugs for marketing. The 1962 Kefaufer–Harris amendments to the Federal Food, Drug and Cosmetic Act require that the FDA consider efficacy as well as safety in the approval of drugs and devices. In addition to the Federal Food, Drug and Cosmetic Act, the legislative base of the FDA includes a number of other statutes, for example, Tea Importation Act, Imported Milk Act, Public Health Service Act (biological products), Fair Packaging and Labeling Act, and Radiation Control for Health and Safety Act. The agency's divisions are:

- Bureau of Biologics
- Bureau of Drugs

---

13. The National Institute of Occupational Safety and Health conducts research and studies and develops standards.

14. Except meat and poultry, which are inspected by the Department of Agriculture.

- Bureau of Foods
- Bureau of Medical Devices
- Bureau of Radiological Health
- Bureau of Veterinary Medicine
- National Center for Toxicological Research

There are ten regional field offices and twenty-two district offices.

Health Resources Administration. This agency is concerned with the planning, development, and distribution of health resources, including manpower planning.

Bureau of Health Facilities. Administers the Hill–Burton program of loans and grants for the construction and modernization of health facilities. Its divisions are:

- Division of Facilities Compliance [15]
- Division of Facilities Conversion and Utilization
- Division of Facilities Financing
- Division of Energy Policy and Programs

Bureau of Health Professions (formerly the Bureau of Health Manpower). Carries out a program of support for health manpower education and training [16] and for research and studies relating to manpower distribution and utilization. It defines and designates *health manpower shortage areas*, which are eligible for assignment of National Health Service Corps personnel and preference for certain grant funds. The Bureau's divisions are:

- Division of Associated Health Professions
- Division of Dentistry
- Division of Nursing

---

15. Responsible for overseeing the requirements that facilities that have received Hill–Burton funding provide services to persons living or employed in their areas ("community services requirement") and that they provide a "reasonable volume" of services to persons unable to pay.

16. Among the grant programs is that for *Area Health Education Centers* (AHECs), regional or state networks for health manpower education, sponsored by designated medical schools. This program was designed to improve (directly and indirectly) access to care by rural and urban underserved communities.

- Division of Medicine
- Division of Health Professions Analysis

Bureau of Health Planning. Primarily responsible for implementing the provisions of the National Health Planning and Resources Development Act of 1974, administering the program of support for state and area health planning and development agencies and activities. Functions include the designation of *health service areas* and the support of corresponding *health systems agencies.* The Bureau's divisions are:

- Division of Regulatory Activities
- Division of Planning Assistance and Assessment
- National Health Planning Information Center

Health Services Administration. This agency is concerned with the provision of health services.

Bureau of Community Health Services. Administers programs related to maternal and child health, family planning, community health centers (neighborhood health centers), migrant health, rural health, and emergency medical services systems. It also includes the *National Health Service Corps,*[17] whose personnel are deployed to areas of particular medical need ("health manpower shortage areas").

Bureau of Medical Services. Administers the medical programs of the Coast Guard and the Bureau of Prisons; a hospital for leprosy patients in Carville, Louisiana; and occupational health services for federal employees. Until recently, it administered eight Public Health Service hospitals and clinics, which cared for merchant seamen, members of the uniformed services, and certain other groups. These facilities are now being taken over by other government agencies or local communities.[18]

---

17. Physicians, dentists, nurse practitioners, nurse midwives, and physicians' assistants.

18. Under the Omnibus Budget Reconciliation Act of 1981. (In 1948 there were twenty-four hospitals. Most were subsequently closed or turned over to local communities. Proposals for closing the remaining eight were long vigorously resisted.)

Indian Health Service. Administers an extensive system of hospitals and health centers that provides health services to American Indians and native Alaskans.

National Institutes of Health. This agency, nominally with the Public Health Service, includes the National Library of Medicine,[19] the Fogarty International Center for the Advanced Study of Health Sciences, and eleven research institutes that carry out and support programs of basic and clinical research. These are:

- National Institute on Aging
- National Cancer Institute
- National Heart, Lung and Blood Institute
- National Institute of Dental Research
- National Institute of Neurological and Communicative Disorders and Stroke
- National Institute of Arthritis, Diabetes and Digestive and Kidney Diseases
- National Institute of Allergy and Infectious Diseases
- National Institute of Child Health and Human Development
- National Institute of General Medical Sciences
- National Eye Institute
- National Institute of Environmental Health Sciences

Office of the Assistant Secretary for Health. The Office of the Assistant Secretary for Health includes, under the direction of the Deputy Assistant Secretary for Health Research, Statistics and Technology, three operating agencies:

National Center for Health Services Research. The Center conducts and supports research and demonstration projects related to the financing, organization, and provision of health care. Special emphasis has been given to the areas of cost, quality, and new types of health manpower.

---

19. The library carries on a wide variety of informational activities, including assistance to medical libraries, support for a Regional Medical Library network, publication of the *Index Medicus*, and development and operation of the computerized Medical Literature and Analysis Retrieval System (MEDLARS). An on-line search service is available via terminals in over 600 institutions. Among available data bases are MEDLINE (MEDLARS On-Line) and TOXLINE (Toxicology Information On-Line).

National Center for Health Statistics.   The Center collects (from state agencies) and reports the official U.S. Vital Statistics. It carries out a program of studies, data evaluation, and methods research relating to the collection and analysis of health data. This includes special periodic surveys, including:

The *Health Interview Survey* — a national household interview study of illness, disability, and health services utilization.[20]

The *Health and Nutrition Examination Survey* — a program of examination and testing of national population samples.

The *Hospital Discharge Survey* — surveys of patient utilization of short stay hospitals.

The *National Ambulatory Medical Care Survey* — was begun in 1973. Data is collected from a sample of practicing physicians.

The *National Nursing Home Survey* — surveys of nursing homes and their residents and staff.

The *Master Facility Inventory* — a listing of all U.S. inpatient health facilities, periodically updated.

The Center is also participating in and provides some grant support for the development of a federal–state–local Cooperative Health Statistics System.

National Center for Health Care Technology.   This center was established in 1978. It has administered a program of studies and evaluations of technological developments in health.

Also among the units of the Office of the Assistant Secretary are the *Office of Health Maintenance Organizations*, which oversees the program of grants for the developments of HMOs, and the *Office of Adolescent Pregnancy Programs.*

Health Care Financing Administration (HCFA)

The newly established Health Care Financing Administration is responsible for the Medicare and Medicaid programs, including quality

20. This was the first system for the regular collection of health related data by the Public Health Service. It was developed under the National Health Survey Act of 1956.

and utilization control. Its divisions are:

Health Standards and Quality Bureau —responsible for the Professional Standards Review Organizations and the certification of Medicare providers.

Bureau of Quality Control —control of fraud and abuse.

Bureau of Program Operations —Medicare and Medicaid in general.

Bureau of Program Policy

The Office of Research, Demonstrations and Statistics carries out and supports Medicare and Medicaid related research and studies. The *Office of Special Programs* oversees the End Stage Renal Disease (ESRD)[21] and Early and Periodic Screening, Diagnosis and Treatment (EPSDT)[22] programs; and special Medicare provisions relating to rural health clinics (reimbursement for nonphysician providers) and group health plans (prepayment).

Social Security Administration (SSA)

The Social Security Administration administers the "social security" program of Old Age, Survivors and Disability Insurance (OASDI) and the program of Supplemental Security Income for the Aged, Blind and Disabled (SSI). It is also responsible for review and authorization of claims for black lung benefits.[23] Subsequent to the 1977 reorganization, it also now administers the federal–state public assistance program of Aid to Families with Dependent Children (AFDC). Program operations are highly decentralized through ten regional offices to some 1,300 local (district and branch) offices. The regional offices and commissioners have the responsibility for liaison and coordination with relevant state and federal agencies.

---

21. Medicare benefits for persons receiving kidney dialysis treatments.
22. A Medicaid mandated screening program for children.
23. Under the Federal Coal Mine Health and Safety Act of 1969.

Office of Human Development Services

The Office of Human Development Services is an umbrella agency for a variety of social services and health related programs for populations deemed to have special needs. Its components are:

Administration on Aging. This agency administers, through state agencies on aging, programs for the elderly under the Older Americans Act.

Administration for Children, Youth and Families. This unit includes the Children's Bureau (which now has responsibility for child welfare services under Title IVB of the Social Security Act), the Head Start Bureau and the Youth Development Bureau.

Administration on Developmental Disabilities.[24] This agency administers a program of services for the developmentally disabled; particularly the mentally retarded.

Administration for Native Americans. This administers a variety of grant programs for Native Americans and their tribal and community organizations (American Indians, Alaskan natives, and native Hawaiians).

HHS Regional Offices

There are ten regional offices of the Department of Health and Human Services, each with a regional director. Their staffs work cooperatively with state and local government and community agencies in carrying out departmental programs. The offices are: I Boston, II New York, III Philadelphia, IV Atlanta, V Chicago, VI Dallas, VII Kansas City, Mo., VIII Denver, IX San Francisco, X Seattle.

INTRODUCTION TO HEALTH LEGISLATION

The many activities of the federal government in health are authorized by the passage of laws, or statutes, by the Congress.

---

24. Mental or physical (neurological) disability first manifested in childhood.

The Enactment of Laws[25]

Proposed legislation, called a *bill*,[26] is introduced in the Senate or House or Representatives by a congressional sponsor.[27] It is assigned a sequential number (e.g., HR-1, S-3) and referred to the appropriate committee for study. Public *hearings* are often held, after which the bill may be amended or entirely redrafted, sometimes in combination with other bills addressed to the same issue. Ultimately, if it is approved, the bill is discharged from the committee with a favorable report and is then placed on the legislative calendar for floor action. A committee does not act on every bill referred to it and there is no time limit within which it must report out a bill.

If passed by the Senate or House (with or without amendments from the floor), the bill is sent to the other chamber where essentially the same process of committee referral, reporting, and floor debate takes place.

If there is substantial disagreement between the two houses on a bill that has been passed by both, *conference committees* will be formed, usually from among the senior members of the committees that reported the bill. If an agreement is arrived at, a *conference report* is made, which is then voted on as a whole, without amendment, by each house. If passed by both houses it is sent to the President for approval. When signed by him, the bill becomes a law or *statute*.

Any legislation that has not been finally passed by both the Senate and House of Representatives by the end of a Congress[28] is dead and must be reintroduced in the next Congress if it is to be again considered. (Only a minority of the many bills introduced in each legislative session become a law.)

The law is then numbered sequentially and by number of the Congress; for example, Public Law 89-97 (PL 89-97) means the 97th

25. This is a general outline of a very complex process.

26. Sometimes legislation is introduced as a *resolution* that has essentially the same practical significance as a bill.

27. Legislation may be drafted by legislators and their staffs by various levels of the Executive Branch or by private citizens or groups. A bill may have a number of congressional sponsors—up to twenty-five in the House and unlimited in the Senate.

28. The two annual sessions spanning the term of office of members of the House of Representatives are known as a Congress. For example, the 92nd Congress extended from January 1971 to December 1972.

law passed by the 89th Congress.[29] The law is printed in pamphlet form known as a *slip law*; later it is published in the *Statutes at Large* and ultimately incorporated into the *United States Code*.

The formal title, which is an integral part of the law, takes the form "An Act to . . ." and may be quite detailed. Often a *short title* is also specified. Frequently, however, a law comes to be known by the names of its chief congressional sponsors. For example, PL 79–725 is formally entitled "An Act to amend the Public Health Service Act to authorize grants to the states for surveying their hospital and public health centers and for planning construction of additional facilities, and to authorize grants to assist in such construction." Its short title is the "Hospital Survey and Construction Act." However, it is generally known as the "Hill–Burton Act" after its sponsors, Senators Lester Hill and Harold Burton.

Occasionally a specific section of an act may be given a specific short title. For example, Title (section) I of PL 92–157 is the *Comprehensive Health Manpower Training Act of 1971*.

Rarely, a law will retain as its popular name its original bill number, notably the *Social Security Amendments of 1972*, which were for a time widely referred to as "HR–1." Sometimes a part of a law will acquire a popular name. For example, the Professional Standards Review Organizations (PSRO) section of the Social Security Amendments of 1972 is often called the "Bennett Amendment" after Senator Wallace Bennett, who amended the original bill with these provisions.

Much legislation is "authorizing" legislation, which establishes or continues programs and authorizes funding for them. *Appropriations bills* actually provide the funds.[30] Often, less is appropriated than has been authorized to be appropriated. Furthermore, the Executive Branch may elect not to spend all the funds appropriated for a particular purpose if these were more than requested or if it does not wish to implement a particular program.

The actual power of the President to "impound" funds appropriated by Congress has been a controversial constitutional question between the legislative and executive branches of the government.

---

29. There is also a series of *private laws* relating to private individuals or claims against the government.

30. Appropriations bills may include other provisions. For example, the "Hyde Amendment" (originally sponsored by Representative Henry J. Hyde), which restricts use of federal funds for abortions, has been added to recent appropriations bills.

This was settled for practical purposes by the *Impoundment Control Act of 1974* whereby the President may temporarily impound funds but must ask the Congress to *rescind* specified appropriations if he wishes not to spend the funds at all. Congress consents by passing *rescission bills*. The President may also *defer* some spending of appropriated funds to the next fiscal year if neither House votes to override the executive order.

If, as has often been the case, an appropriations committee fails to pass a bill authorizing new funds for the relevant executive departments, a *continuing resolution* is passed that authorizes spending at the previous year's levels for a limited period of time.

Congressional Budget Process

With the passage of the Budget Control Act of 1974 the congressional budget process has been extensively revised and strengthened. (Previously, the congressional "budget" consisted essentially of the independent actions of the various authorizing and appropriations committees.) The process is very complex. In brief, under the new procedures, a preliminary budget resolution is developed in the spring by the House and Senate budget committees and passed in the usual way by both houses. This resolution sets general spending targets for some nineteen broad categories of governmental funding. A complete *reconciliation* process involving the authorization and budget committee may then be carried out, resulting in a reconciliation bill.[31] A second, binding budget resolution is passed in the fall, in theory before the beginning of the fiscal year.[32] A third budget resolution may be required during the fiscal year to accommodate needed supplementary appropriations.

Regulations

Many of the details of the various laws are left to be spelled out in *regulations*[33] prescribed by the various administrative agencies of the

31. This mechanism was first used in 1980.

32. Until 1976, the fiscal year (FY) ran from July 1 to June 30. It was then changed to run from October 1 to September 30, to allow more time for the budget and appropriations process. FY 1982, for example, is October 1, 1981 to September 30, 1982.

33. The phrase "rules and regulations" is sometimes used. *Rules* is a technical term for regulations; the process of developing regulations is sometimes called *rulemaking*.

Executive Branch. As these are made, they are published in the *Federal Register*, taking effect thirty days thereafter. (Often these are published as proposed regulations, which are then revised after comments have been received from interested parties.) These regulations are then incorporated in the *Code of Federal Regulations* and have the force of law.

Congressional Committees

There are sixteen standing committees in the Senate and twenty-two in the House of Representatives, most of which have several subcommittees that address bills in detail, hold hearings, and issue reports to the full committee. There are also several special or select committees, considered to be temporary, which have been established to study special problems (e.g., House Select Committee on Aging, Senate Special Committee on Aging).

Many committees are involved in matters related to health but those of particular importance are:

House Ways and Means Committee. Jurisdiction includes social security (Social Security Subcommittee) and Medicare (*Health Subcommittee*). The special importance of Ways and Means derives from the constitutional provision that laws raising revenue must originate in the House of Representatives. Such (tax) measures are assigned to this committee.

Senate Finance Committee. Jurisdiction includes Medicare and Medicaid (*Health Subcommittee*).

House Energy and Commerce Committee. Jurisdiction includes most health legislation including Medicaid (*Subcommittee on Health and the Environment*).

Senate Labor and Human Resources Committee. Jurisdiction includes health legislation in general. Medicare and Medicaid issues are also addressed in cooperation with the Senate Finance Committee.

House and Senate Appropriations Committees. Subcommittees for Labor, Health and Human Services, and Education appropriate funds for these departments.

Grants-in-Aid

Many of the funds distributed to the states and localities under federal legislation are made available by the mechanism of *grants-in-aid*. These grants are authorized in the various federal laws for stated purposes and are given to the states and to local organizations, agencies, and individuals, under certain conditions and in accordance with certain regulations.

Formula grants. Funds are allotted by a formula that takes into consideration such factors as state population, per capita income, and the extent of health problems.

Matching grants. Funds must be matched up to a specified percentage by the state, agency, or institution receiving the grant.

Research grants. Funds are granted competitively to individuals, agencies, and institutions to carry out specific research work outlined in research proposals submitted by the applicants.

Training grants. Funds are granted competitively to institutions engaged in certain health manpower training activities. These may include student stipends.

Capitation grants. Funds are allotted to educational institutions by formulas related to student enrollment.

Grants-in-aid to the states are usually made from allotments among the states in accordance with the specified formula. These grants also carry such requirements as the submission of a *state plan* concerning the problem or purpose in question, assignment of the responsibility for administration of the plan to a *single state agency* and conformation to guidelines and standards regarding use of the funds. They are typically formula grants, and generally have matching requirements.

Programs of grants-in-aid are usually authorized for stipulated periods of time only, usually two to five years; these authorizations must be renewed periodically if programs are to continue. Thus, at any one time, several of these will be in various stages of the legislative process, for continuation and amendment.[34]

In recent years federal agencies have made considerable use of the *contract* mechanism for funding health-related research, studies, and other activities. "Requests for proposals" (RFPs) are circulated by the funding agency to institutions, agencies, and individuals active in the area of the proposed work.

Categorical grants are made for relatively narrowly defined categories of problems, that is, entities such as communicable disease, family planning, and maternal and child health.

Block Grants are for more broadly defined purposes and permit more discretion in use of the funds by the states and with less specific federal regulation. Frequent proposals have been made for further consolidation of categorical grant programs into block grants in keeping with the trend toward decreasing federal regulation and facilitating more decisionmaking at the state and local levels ("new federalism"). A major such step was taken under the 1981 *Omnibus Budget Reconciliation Act* among whose many provisions was the consolidation of fifty-seven categorical grant programs for health, education, community development, and welfare into nine block grants, including four for health programs.

Revenue Sharing

The concept of *revenue sharing* has been advocated as a more appropriate mechanism for financial aid to the states than the relatively categorical approach of the grant-in-aid programs. The first revenue sharing legislation was passed in 1972, under the State and Local Fiscal Assistance Act of 1972. Funds were allocated to state governments with relatively few restrictions and to local governments for "priority expenditures" (necessary capital expenditures, and operating expenses in the areas of public safety, environmental protection, public transportation, health, recreation, libraries, social services for the poor and aged, and financial administration). The states have now been excluded at least temporarily from the program, which has remained controversial.

---

34. One exception is the research and training grants of The National Institutes of Health, which have no statutory time limit though subject to the usual appropriations bills.

Congressional Support Offices

General Accounting Office. The General Accounting Office under the direction of the Comptroller General is an independent agency within the legislative branch. It assists the Congress directly and by carrying out review and auditing of programs and activities authorized by Congress, and makes recommendations designed to make government operations more efficient and effective. It prescribes the accounting principles and standards to be followed by federal agencies, and makes determinations as to the legality of actions taken in the use of public funds.

Office of Technology Assessment. This office was established in 1972 to study and advise the Congress about issues related to the application of technology. Its activities include cost-effectiveness and cost–benefit analyses of medical and health procedures and technologies.

Congressional Budget Office. This office was established by the Congressional Budget and Impoundment Act of 1974. It carries out studies and analyses relating to fiscal policies and the federal budget.

Specific Health Legislation

The following sections summarize the principal federal legislation related to health care. They are organized in such a way as to give a general sense of the historical development of these laws. They do not attempt to deal with the complex political, social, and economic background of this body of legislation, nor with its implementation and impact; they are designed to provide a base from which to address these issues.

The Social Security Act, and the Public Health Service Act are described in particular detail, as they have been the vehicles for such important programs as Medicare and Medicaid and the Hill–Burton health planning and health manpower programs.

THE SOCIAL SECURITY ACT (1935)

An Act to provide for the general welfare by establishing a system of federal old age benefits, and by enabling the several States to make more adequate provision for aged persons, blind persons, dependent and crippled children, maternal and child welfare, public health, and the administration of their unemployment compensation laws; to establish a Social Security Board: to raise revenue; and for other purposes.

The Social Security Act of 1935 was a landmark piece of legislation, which was developed and passed during the Great Depression. It represented the first major entrance of the federal government into the area of social insurance and it greatly and significantly expanded federal grant-in-aid assistance to the states. It has formed the base for important federal programs in health including, most recently, Medicare and Medicaid. Its eleven titles (divisions) are summarized in Appendix D.

The act established the "Social Security" program of old age benefits (Title I); provided for federal financial assistance to the states' public assistance ("welfare") programs for the needy elderly, dependent children, and the blind; provided fiscal incentives for the establishment of state unemployment funds; and established financial assistance for maternal and child health and child welfare services (Title V) and greatly increased assistance for state and local public health programs.

AMENDMENTS TO THE SOCIAL SECURITY ACT, 1939-1963

In the ensuing years, there have been many amendments to the original Social Security Act, enlarging gradually the scope of its provisions. The following are especially noteworthy:

Social Security Amendments of 1939. Benefits for dependents and survivors were added to the old age social security program.

Social Security Amendments of 1950. The program of federal aid to state public assistance programs was extended to permanently and totally disabled persons under a new Title XIV. Federal matching for state payments to providers of medical services to persons on public assistance (*vendor payments*) was also added. The "federally aided public assistance categories" established under the Social Security Act (initially and as amended) were now:

- Old Age Assistance (OAA)
- Aid to Families with Dependent Children (AFDC)
- Aid to the Blind (AB)
- Aid to the Permanently and Totally Disabled (APTD)

Social Security Amendments of 1956. A program of benefits for eligible disabled persons was added to the social security program, now known as Old Age, Survivors and Disability Insurance (OASDI).

Social Security Amendments of 1960 ("Kerr–Mills" Act). The most important provisions of the 1960 amendments were those related to medical services for the aged, provisions that were passed after extensive congressional debate concerning health insurance for the aged.

Title I of the Social Security Act was amended to read *Grants to the States for Old Age Assistance and Medical Assistance for the Aged*: ". . . for the purpose of enabling each state to furnish medical assistance on behalf of aged individuals who are not recipients of old age assistance but whose income and resources are insufficient to meet the costs of necessary medical services. . . ."

This established a new program of *medical assistance for the aged* (MAA) providing for federal aid to the states for payments for medical care for "medically indigent" persons age sixty-five and over.

As with all grants-in-aid, participation by the states was optional. A broad range of medical services could be made available to the recipients with the stipulation that these include at least some institutional and some noninstitutional care. The federal participation was 50 to 83 percent of costs according to per capita income in the state. A total of twenty-five states implemented this "Kerr–Mills program," which was the forerunner of Medicaid.

Maternal and Child Health and Mental Retardation Planning Amendments of 1963. These amendments were "to assist states and communities in preventing and combating mental retardation through expansion and improvement of the maternal and child health and crippled children's programs, through provision of prenatal, maternity, and infant care for individuals with conditions associated with childbearing that may lead to mental retardation, and through planning for comprehensive action to combat mental retardation." A number of additions were made to Title V, including *special project grants for maternity and infant care* for low income mothers and infants and grants for *research projects* related to maternal and child health and crippled children's services. A new grants program was also added: Title *XVII, Grants for Planning Comprehensive Action To Combat Mental Retardation.*[35]

SOCIAL SECURITY AMENDMENTS OF 1965 (MEDICARE, MEDICAID, AND CHILD HEALTH AMENDMENTS)

The Social Security amendments of 1965 established the national program of health insurance for the aged now known as "Medicare."[36] It was the culmination of many years of national and congressional debate and is of great historic importance. The amendments also included provisions for expansion of the Kerr–Mills medical assistance program to groups other than the elderly—a program now known as "Medicaid." Significant additions were made to Title V, and changes were also made in the OASDI and Public Assistance titles of the Social Security Act.

Health Insurance for the Aged (Medicare)

Title XVIII, *Health Insurance for the Aged*, was added to the Social Security Act.

Part A: Hospital Insurance Benefits. This insurance program provides basic protection against the costs of hospital and related posthospital services. This was to be financed by an increase in the Social Security earnings tax (payroll tax). Benefits included:

- *Inpatient hospital* services for up to 90 days during any spell of illness and psychiatric inpatient services for up to 190 days in a lifetime.

---

35. This provision for planning grants has since expired.

36. This term was originally applied to the program for medical care for servicemen's dependents under the Dependents Medical Care Act (1956). It is now universally applied to this program of health insurance for the aged.

- Posthospital *extended care* services for up to 100 days during any spell of illness.
- Posthospital *home health* services for up to 100 visits in a one-year period.
- Hospital outpatient *diagnostic* services.

Part B: Supplemental Medical Insurance Benefits. This is a voluntary insurance program financed from premium payments by enrollees with matching payments from general revenues. Benefits included:

- *Physicians' services* and related services such as x-rays and laboratory tests and supplies and equipment.
- *Home health services.*

There are provisions for cost sharing by beneficiaries (deductibles and coinsurance) and for claims and payments to be handled by *fiscal intermediaries* (Part A) and *carriers* (Part B).[37] Institutional providers may participate by complying with *conditions of participation*; these include, for hospitals and nursing homes, procedures for *utilization review.* Because of the importance of this legislation, an extensive summary of the original provisions is set forth in Appendix E.

Federal–State Medical Assistance Program (Medicaid)

Title XIX, *Grants to the States for Medical Assistance Programs*, was added to the Social Security Act.

This title established a single program of medical assistance for public assistance recipients, and extended eligibility to medically indigent persons not on welfare. It is a federal–state matching grant program, and replaced the Kerr–Mills program for the medically indigent elderly.

Under this program, states were to provide at least some of each of five basic services:

- Inpatient hospital services
- Outpatient hospital services
- Other laboratory and x-ray services

---

37. Despite the differing terminology, both fiscal intermediaries and "carriers" are generally area Blue Cross and Blue Shield plans and insurance companies.

- Skilled nursing home services
- Physicians' services

A wide spectrum of additional services could also be made available by the states. The federal share of the program's costs is 50 to 83 percent, according to a state's per capita income.

For a more detailed summary of this title (as originally enacted), see Appendix E.

Maternal and Child Health Services

There were a number of amendments to Title V. (See Appendix E.) Most notable was the provision for special project grants for comprehensive services for *children and youth.* These children and youth (C&Y) projects and the maternal and infant care (M&I) projects developed under the 1963 amendments have formed the core services of many neighborhood health centers.

SOCIAL SECURITY AMENDMENTS, 1966–1971

During 1966 and 1967 there were several short amendments to the Medicare section of the Social Security Act, providing for extension of the initial and first general enrollment periods, and adjusting the reimbursement formula for proprietary extended care facilities.

Social Security Amendments of 1967

These extensive amendments included a number of changes and adjustments in the Medicare and Medicaid programs. Among these are the following:

Medicare Amendments

- Elimination of the requirement that a physician *certify* to the medical necessity of admissions to general hospitals and of outpatient hospital services (the requirement for periodic certification after admission remains).
- Inclusion under Part B of the services of *podiatrists* for nonroutine foot care.

- Transfer of hospital *outpatient diagnostic services* from Part A to Part B.

- Provision for the payment of *full reasonable charges for radiologists' and pathologists' services* to inpatients (deductible and coinsurance no longer applicable to these services).

- Provision for purchase of durable medical equipment for use in the home.

- Inclusion of outpatient *physical therapy* under Part B.

- Provision for payment under Part B for *diagnostic x-rays* taken in a patient's home or nursing home.

- Addition of a *lifetime reserve of sixty days* of coverage for inpatient hospital care (coinsurance of one-half the inpatient deductible).

Medicaid Amendments

- Provision for *limitation of federal participation* in medical assistance payments to families whose income does not exceed 133 percent of the income limit for AFDC payments in any state.

- For the medically indigent, the states could select the "basic five" services or seven out of the first fourteen of the services listed under the original legislation. The states must continue to provide the "basic five" services for public assistance recipients.

- Requirement, as of July 1969, that the states provide health screening services for Medicaid eligible children and such corrective measures as provided in regulations.

- If nursing home or hospital services are selected, physicians' services in these institutions are also to be included.

- Provision that persons covered under medical assistance will have free choice of qualified medical facilities and practitioners.

- Requirements that skilled nursing homes providing services under the medical assistance program meet the requirements for state licensure, and meet standards similar to those applicable to extended care facilities; that their administrators be licensed; and that there be a program of regular medical review of care furnished.

Maternal and Child Health Amendments[38]

- Revised Title V to consolidate all its programs for maternal and child health and crippled children under one authorization.
- Continued for a limited period provisions for the special projects for maternal and infant care and children and youth (ultimately to be included under the formula grant program) and added authorization for special projects for dental health of children.
- Made special provision for funding of family planning services.
- Continued and expanded provisions for training of personnel, and added authorization for research projects related to maternal and child health and crippled children's services.
- Transferred authorization for child welfare services to Title IV.

A provision was also included for federal participation in payment for services in *intermediate care* facilities[39] for public assistance recipients.

In 1969, a rider was added to an unrelated bill (PL 91-55) providing for additional modifications of the Medicaid program:

- Extension to July 1, 1977 of the deadline for states to establish comprehensive medical assistance programs.
- The states are permitted to reduce some medical services previously available under their medical assistance programs (but prohibiting reduction of cash payments to public assistance recipients).

An additional amendment in 1971 (PL 92-223) broadened the intermediate care facilities provisions to include, optionally, Medicaid recipients other than those on public assistance.

---

38. Child Health Act of 1967.

39. An institution providing a level of care beyond room and board, but not of a degree required of a skilled nursing home.

SOCIAL SECURITY AMENDMENTS OF 1972

The Social Security Amendments of 1972 made important changes in the Social Security Act, including extensive amendments of the Medicare and Medicaid provisions.

Provisions Relating to Medicare and Medicaid

There were a large number of amendments (ninety-seven separate sections) affecting Medicare and Medicaid, many addressed to the control of costs, many making significant changes. Notable among the provisions are the following, briefly summarized:

Health insurance for the disabled.   Persons who have received cash benefits under the disability insurance provisions of the Social Security Act for at least twenty-four months will be eligible for medical benefits under Title XVIII of the Social Security Act (which will now read *Health Insurance for the Aged and Disabled*).

Part B. Premiums, Deductibles and Automatic Enrollment. Part B premiums will not be increased more than the most recent percentage increase in social security cash benefits. Beneficiaries will be automatically enrolled upon entitlement with provision made for those who wish to decline enrollment. The annual deductible is increased to $60.

Cost sharing under Medicaid. (1) The states must charge an income-related enrollment fee to medically indigent persons included under Medicaid programs, and may charge nominal deductibles and copayments; (2) The states may charge public assistance recipients nominal deductibles and copayments for other than the basic mandated services.

Deferred loss of Medicaid due to increased earnings. Families who lose Medicaid eligibility because of increased earnings will remain covered for four months.

Limitation of payments for unnecessary capital expenditures. Payment will not be made for capital expenditures that have been disapproved by state or local planning agencies.

Experiments and demonstrations related to increased economy and efficiency of health services. Grants and contracts are authorized for studies, experiments, and demonstrations related to prospective reimbursement; the three-day hospitalization requirement for skilled nursing home admission; ambulatory surgical centers, intermediate care facilities; home health and day care services; payment for services of physician's assistants and nurse practitioners; and use of clinical psychologists.

Health Maintenance Organizations (HMOs). Single annual per capita payments may be made to health maintenance organizations for Part A and Part B services provided to or arranged for Medicare beneficiaries. Such organizations must provide care to a group of enrollees of whom at least one half are not Medicare beneficiaries. Up to 20 percent of any savings made by a health maintenance organization relative to the per capita annual costs of services to non-HMO enrollees will be divided equally between the organization and the Medicare trust funds.

Payment of teaching physicians. Payments under Part B for services of physicians in hospital teaching programs will generally be made on a cost basis only, except for bona fide private patients. Payment for donated services of such physicians will be made to a fund designated for charitable or educational purposes.[40]

Advance approval of skilled nursing facility and home health benefits. Minimum periods of presumed eligibility for posthospital services may be established by the Secretary.[41]

Elimination of requirement of progressively more comprehensive Medicaid programs. The Title IX section requiring that the states progress toward the provision of comprehensive Medicaid services by July 1, 1977 is repealed.

Level of state Medicaid funding. The Title IX section prohibiting a state from reducing its aggregate payments for Medicaid services is repealed.

Payments to states for claims and information systems. Matching funds may be paid to the states for development and installation of claims processing and information retrieval systems (90 percent of costs) and, under certain conditions, for their operation (75 percent of costs).

---

40. Implementation was subsequently posponed.
41. Addressed the issue of retroactive denial of benefits.

Utilization review under Medicaid. Hospitals and skilled nursing facilities participating in Medicaid or child health programs must, with some exceptions, use the same utilization review committees as are used under the Medicare program.

Validation of Joint Commission on Accreditation of Hospitals surveys. Arrangements are authorized for the state Medicare certifying agencies to survey, by sampling, participating hospitals that have been accredited by the Joint Commission on Accreditation of Hospitals. The Secretary may in addition prescribe higher standards than required by accreditation by the Commission.

Conformation of skilled care services and facilities under Medicare and Medicaid. Skilled care services are similarly defined with respect to both Medicare and Medicaid, and standards of skilled nursing facilities are to be the same under both programs. The term *extended care facility* is eliminated.

Professional Standards Review. This is the most extensive and important of the provisions directed to the problems of cost and quality control and medical necessity of services.[42] A new part (B) *Professional Standards Review* is added to Title XI of the Social Security Act. Provision is made for the establishment of *Professional Standards Review Organizations* within states for the review of the professional activities of physicians and other practitioners, and institutional and other providers of services in designated geographical areas. The review of services provided other than in institutions will be at the option of the organization and subject to the approval of the Secretary. These organizations are to be associations of physicians and open to and representative of physicians in the area. (After January 1, 1976, and then only if there is no such organization meeting the specified conditions, other competent agencies or organizations may be designated.) Statewide Professional Standards Review Councils and a National Professional Standards Review Council are also to be established.

---

42. The declared purpose of this section is to assure "that the services for which payment may be made under the Social Security Act will conform to appropriate professional standards and that payment for such services will be made (1) only when, and to the extent, medically necessary . . ."; and (2) in the case of inpatient services, only when these cannot "effectively be provided on an outpatient basis or more economically in a health care facility of a different type."

Social services in skilled nursing facilities. It is no longer to be required under Medicare that medical social services be furnished in a skilled nursing facility.

Chiropractic services. Chiropractors' services are covered under Medicare and Medicaid with respect to treatment by means of manual manipulation of the spine; in the case of Medicare, this is specifically to be for correction of a subluxation demonstrated by x-ray.

Speech pathology services. Speech pathology is covered as a part of outpatient physical therapy services under Medicare.

Review of care in intermediate care facilities. The requirements for professional review of care and placement of patients are extended to intermediate care facilities.

Public information concerning survey reports. The pertinent findings of surveys of health care institutions and agencies with regard to compliance with conditions of participation under Medicare are to be made available to the public.

Family planning services. Family planning services are added to the basic services that must be made available under Medicaid.

Penalty for failure to provide child health screening under Medicaid. The matching funds to the states under Medicaid will be reduced by 1 percent where the states do not implement the previous requirements for providing for child health screening and subsequent corrective treatment services for children in families receiving aid for dependent children.[43]

Home health services coinsurance. Coinsurance payments for home health services under Part B are eliminated.

Treatment for chronic renal disease. Persons insured under Social Security, and their dependents, who require hemodialysis or renal transplantation for chronic renal disease are deemed disabled for purpose of coverage under Title XVIII, beginning three months after initiation of a course of renal dialysis. Reimbursement is to be limited to treatment centers meeting specified requirements.

---

43. The programs established under these provisions have come to be known as Early and Periodic Screening, Diagnosis and Treatment (EPSDT) programs.

Supplemental Security Income for the Aged, Blind, and Disabled

This amendment created, effective January 1, 1974, a new federal minimum income program, Supplemental Security Income (SSI) (under a new Title XVI) to replace the federally aided adult public assistance programs. Grants to the states for social services for these groups were continued under a new Title VI. (No change is made in the federal-state programs of aid to families with dependent children.)

SOCIAL SECURITY AMENDMENTS, 1974-1981

Social Services Amendments of 1974

The purpose of these amendments was to consolidate previous federal-state social service programs in a block grant that would incorporate a ceiling on federal matching funds while providing reasonable flexibility to the states in determining services to be provided and reduction of the federal regulatory role. A new Title XX, *Grants to the States for Services*, was added to the Social Security Act. Stated goals of the program included the prevention and remedy of neglect, abuse, or exploitation of children or adults and the preservation of families, and the prevention of inappropriate institutional care through community based programs. A wide spectrum of social services could be provided including, for example, child care services; protective, foster, and day care services for children and adults; counseling; family planning services; homemaker services; and home delivered meals. Services could be made available to persons with incomes of up to 115 percent of the state median but 50 percent of federal expenditures were to be on behalf of recipients of public assistance, Aid to Families with Dependent Children, Supplemental Security Income, or Medicaid. Provisions also required public notice of a state plan for services and opportunity for comment by the public. Other provisions provided for the establishment or expansion of state programs (under Aid to Families with Dependent Children) for locating absent parents, establishing paternity, and obtaining child support.

Medicare-Medicaid Antifraud and Abuse Amendments (1977)

These amendments incorporated a large number of provisions directed toward program monitoring, the prevention and detection of fraud and abuse, and cost containment. They included the strengthening of criminal and other penalties, adjustments in the professional standards review program, including clarification of the relationship between the PSROs and the state Medicaid agencies, increased funding for the establishment of state Medicaid fraud control units, and provisions for the establishment of uniform reporting systems for hospitals and other health care institutions and organizations.

Rural Health Clinic Services Amendments (1977)

This legislation provided that rural health clinics without physicians routinely on site, located in medically underserved areas, and meeting specific requirements, could be reimbursed under Medicare and Medicaid for services provided by nurse practitioners and physician's assistants. Arrangements were required whereby one or more physicans would be available for supervision and guidance, for review of services provided, and for patient referral where required. Demonstration projects were authorized for reimbursement for services by these personnel in clinics in urban underserved areas.

Medicare Endstage Renal Disease Amendments (1978)

These amendments made a number of adjustments in the Medicare renal disease program (reimbursement for renal dialysis and renal transplantation for chronic renal disease) directed particularly toward control of its costs. Reimbursement incentives were added to encourage the use of home dialysis and renal transplantation, a variety of reimbursement methods for renal dialysis facilities were authorized as were studies relating to end stage renal disease, including those related to cost reduction. The Secretary of Health, Education and Welfare was explicitly authorized to establish renal disease network areas and network coordinating councils, with some patient representation, for program planning and review.

Medicare and Medicaid Amendments of 1980[44]

This legislation made numerous technical and other amendments to the Medicare/Medicaid program (fifty-seven separate sections), many reflecting continuing concern with cost containment and cost efficiency. Among the provisions were the authorization for small rural hospitals to use their beds on a "swing" basis as acute or long-term beds as needed, and for "swing-bed" demonstration projects for large and urban hospitals. Further adjustments were made in the PSRO program. The *home health services* provisions were revised to remove the 100 visit/year limit for both Part A and Part B, to eliminate the required three-day hospital stay for visits under Part A, and the deductible under Part B. The need for occupational therapy was made one of the possible qualifying criteria for initial eligibility for such visits. The previous provision that proprietary home health agencies could participate in Medicare only in states that licensed home health agencies was eliminated. *Alcohol detoxification facility services* were added to benefits under Part A. The provision of the 1972 amendments relating to payments of *supervising physicians in teaching hospitals* (Section 227, the implementation of which had been postponed) was modified to provide for payment of such physicians under Part B and making explicit the level of patient care responsibility that must be assumed by these attending physicians for such reimbursement. State Medicaid programs were required to provide payment for services by *nurse–midwives* (services they are legally authorized by the state to perform).

Medicare and Medicaid Amendments of 1981[45]

These amendments (forty-six sections), passed in the context of extensive federal budget reductions, particularly addressed the reduction of program costs. Coverage of alcohol detoxification facility services was eliminated as was occupational therapy as a basis for initial entitlement to home health services. The Part B deductible was increased to $75.

---

44. Title IX of the Omnibus Reconciliation Act of 1980.
45. Title XXI, Subtitles A, B, C of the Omnibus Budget Reconciliation Act of 1981.

The Secretary of Health and Human Services was directed to assess the relative performance of the professional standard review organizations, with the number of PSROs whose funding agreements could be terminated by the end of fiscal year (FY) 1982 limited to not more than 30 percent of current PSROs; the use of PSROs by state Medicaid agencies was made optional. Matching federal Medicaid payments to the states were to be reduced by percentages of the amounts to which the states would otherwise be entitled: the 3 percent in FY 1982, 4 percent in FY 1983, and 4.5 percent in FY 1984. Each state's reduction could be lowered by 1 percent for each of three conditions: operation of a qualified hospital cost review program, an unemployment rate over 15 percent of the national average, and a specific amount of fraud and abuse recovery.

All previous coverage requirements for the medically needy were repealed, except that home health services must continue to be made available to persons eligible for skilled nursing facility care. If any medically needy groups were to be covered, new minimum requirements were established including ambulatory services for children, prenatal and delivery services for pregnant women, and ambulatory services for groups covered for institutional services.

Certain additional waivers of the "freedom of choice" of provider by Medicaid beneficiaries are authorized. (Previously waivers were authorized to permit a state to conduct special experimental or demonstration projects.) In addition, states may "lock in" beneficiaries who overutilize services to a particular provider for a reasonable time period. States may purchase laboratory services and medical devices by competitive bidding. A state may, by waiver, be allowed to include under Medicaid nonmedical home or community services to persons who would otherwise require care in a nursing home.

Maternal and Child Health Block Grant Act (1981)[46]

These amendments consolidated seven grant programs from Title V of the Social Security Act and from the Public Health Service Act into a block grant under a new Title V: *Maternal and Child Health Services Block Grant*. The consolidated programs are the maternal and child health and crippled children's programs, genetic disease re-

---

46. Title XXI, Subtitle D, Omnibus Budget Reconciliation Act of 1981.

search, adolescent pregnancy services, sudden infant death syndrome research, hemophilia research, Supplemental Security Income (SSI) payments to crippled children, and lead-based poisoning research.

SUMMARY OF MEDICARE AND MEDICAID

Title XVIII. Health Insurance for the Aged and Disabled (Medicare)

Part A. Hospital Insurance

Benefits.   Part A benefits include:

Hospital inpatient services

- Up to ninety days during any spell of illness.[47] Deductible and coinsurance after the sixtieth hospital day.
- Lifetime reserve—sixty days (coinsurance).
- Lifetime limit for inpatient psychiatric care—190 days.

Posthospital extended care services

- Up to 100 days in a skilled nursing facility during any spell of illness. Coinsurance after the twentieth day.
- Three-day prior hospital admission required.
- Continuing *skilled nursing care* or other skilled rehabilitation services must be needed for a condition for which the preceding inpatient services were received.

Posthospital home health services

- Skilled nursing care or physical or speech therapy must be needed. Services are to be rendered under a plan established and periodically reviewed by a physician.

Exclusions.   Excluded are private duty nurses and the cost of the first three pints of blood.

Financing.   Part A is financed by an additional social security tax on employees, employers, and self-employed persons.

---

47. Also referred to as a "benefit period."

Conditions of Participation. Conditions of participation include utilization review plans for hospitals, skilled nursing facilities, and home health agencies.

Part B. Supplementary Medical Insurance

Benefits. Part B benefits include:

Physicians' services

- Services of doctors of medicine and osteopathy, including professional services of hospital-based specialists (radiologists and pathologists).
- Limited, specified services by dentists, podiatrists, optometrists, and chiropractors.

Hospital outpatient services

Diagnostic procedures (e.g., laboratory and x-ray services)

Home health services

Outpatient physical therapy and speech pathology services

Other medical and health services

- Supplies, equipment, prostheses, radiation therapy, ambulance services (only, and under limited conditions for transportation to a hospital or skilled nursing facility).
- Renal dialysis services.
- Rural health clinic services (under specified conditions).

Deductibles and Coinsurance. Deductible is $75 per year; coinsurance is 20 percent of charges. (No deductible or coinsurance for home health services or radiologists' and pathologists' services to inpatients.)

Exclusions. These include glasses, dentures, hearing aids, drugs, check-ups, dental care, routine foot care. There is a $250 annual limit on out-of-hospital psychiatric services.

Financing. Part B is financed by a monthly premium plus government matching.

Administration.   Health Care Financing Administration.

Title XIX.   Grants to States for Medical Assistance Programs (Medicaid)

Federal matching grants are made available, at the option of the states, for medical assistance programs for:

- Recipients of federally aided public assistance (Aid to Families with Dependent Children, AFDC).[48]
- Recipients of Supplemental Security Income benefits (SSI).
- Medically indigent in comparable groups (families with dependent children, as defined for purposes of public assistance, and the aged, blind, and disabled).
- Other needy children.

Programs for AFDC and SSI recipients are to include (some of each of) five basic services:

- Inhospital services
- Outpatient hospital services
- Other laboratory and x-ray services
- Skilled nursing home services
- Physicians' services

Also to be included by each participating state are:

- A program for screening of eligible children for defects and chronic conditions, and appropriate treatment (Early and Periodic Screening, Diagnosis and Treatment, EPSDT).
- Family planning services.

The states may also optionally include virtually any additional medical care services.

---

48. Prior to January 1, 1974, the federally aided public assistance groups ("welfare") also included the indigent aged, blind, and disabled. Under the 1972 Social Security amendments, the latter three groups are now under the federal Supplemental Security Income program.

Federal matching is 50 to 83 percent of costs (according to state's per capita income).

All states except Arizona have established Medicaid programs.

Administration. Health Care Financing Administration. The administering state agency is usually the department of public welfare.

THE PUBLIC HEALTH SERVICE ACT

> An Act to consolidate and revise the laws relating to the Public Health Service and for other purposes."

The Public Health Service Act of 1944 revised and brought together in one statute all existing legislation concerning the Public Health Service (including Title VI of the Social Security Act). It set forth provisions for the organization, staffing, and activities of the Service. It has subsequently been the vehicle, by amendment, of a number of important federal grant-in-aid programs. The following is a brief summary of its major provisions.

Title I. Short Title and Definitions

Title II. Administration

The general organization of the Public Health Service is set forth, to be administered by the Surgeon General under the direction of the Federal Security Administrator. The Service shall consist of the Office of the Surgeon General, the National Institute of Health, the Bureau of Medical Services, and the Bureau of State Services.

Grades, ranks, and titles of the Commissioned Corps, and relevant policies and regulations are specified. Commissioned officers include personnel in "medicine, surgery, dentistry, hygiene, sanitary engineering, pharmacy, nursing, or related scientific specialties in public health."

Title III. General Powers and Duties
of the Public Health Service

Part A. Research and Investigations. The service shall conduct, encourage, cooperate in, and promote research and investigations relating to physical and mental diseases and impairments.

Activities shall include studies and investigations regarding the use and misuse of narcotic drugs. The Surgeon General shall give aid and advice to state officials in the care, treatment, and rehabilitation of narcotics addicts.

Part B. Federal–State Cooperation. The Surgeon General is authorized to provide *assistance to state and local authorities* in prevention and control of communicable diseases.

A health conference of the state health authorities shall be called annually.[49] Provision is made for the collection and compilation of *vital statistics.*

Section 314 provides for grants and services to the states to assist in *venereal disease control, tuberculosis control*, and the establishment and maintenance of adequate *state and local public health services.* Annual allotments to the states shall be made on the basis of population, the size of the venereal disease and tuberculosis problems and other special health problems, and the financial need of the respective states. Grants shall be paid on the condition that the states spend for the same general purpose from its funds an amount determined in accordance with regulations.

The Surgeon General shall issue from time to time *information related to public health*, including publications for the public, weekly reports on health conditions, and other pertinent information for those engaged in work related to the functions of the Service.

Part C. Hospitals, Medical Examinations, and Medical Care. The management and operation of the institutions, hospitals, and stations of the Service is set forth. Medical care is to be provided for *merchant seamen* and certain other persons including members of the U.S. Maritime Service, Merchant Marine cadets, and quarantine and immigration detainees. The Service is to furnish medical services in

---

49. Known as the Conference of State and Territorial Health Officers.

penal and correctional institutions of the United States. The Surgeon General is authorized to provide medical services to *federal employees* for work-related illness or injury and medical examinations for employees and retirees. Medical examination of *aliens* is provided for. Members of the Coast Guard, Coast and Geodetic Survey, and the Commissioned Corps of the Public Health Service are entitled to treatment and hospitalization by the Service.

Part D. Lepers. The Public Health Service shall receive and care for persons with leprosy.

Part E. Narcotics Addicts. Care and treatment, in hospitals of the Service, of narcotics addicts who are federal prisoners or who voluntarily request treatment.

Part F. Biological Products. Regulation of the manufacture, labeling, and sale of biological products (virus, serum, toxin, antitoxin, or other product) applicable to the prevention or cure of disease or injuries.

Part G. Quarantine and Inspection. Inspection, quarantine, and other procedures necessary to prevent transmission or spread of communicable diseases from foreign countries into states or possessions, or from one state or possession into another.

Title IV. National Cancer Institute

The National Cancer Institute shall be a division of the National Institute of Health, to carry out the purposes of Part A of Title III (Research and Investigation) with regard to cancer. It is to conduct and assist researches, investigations, and studies relating to the cause, prevention and treatment of cancer; provide training and instruction relating to diagnoses and treatment of cancer; and provide fellowships in the Institute.

Grants-in-aid for cancer projects shall be made only after review and recommendations of the National Cancer Advisory Council.

Title V. Miscellaneous

Miscellaneous regulations, and authorization for the *admission to St. Elizabeths Hospital* of insane patients entitled to treatment by the Service.

Amendments to the Public Health Service Act

There have been many amendments to the Public Health Service Act. Many were major pieces of legislation, which have in turn been much amended. The following amendments are particularly noteworthy; several of these (denoted with an asterisk) are described more fully in subsequent sections.

*Hospital Survey and Construction Act of 1946 (Hill–Burton Act). This inaugurated the Hill–Burton program of health facilities construction.

*Health Amendments of 1956 (Grants for Training in Public Health and Nursing). These initiated the program of federal assistance for education and training of health personnel, which has been gradually extended and broadened by subsequent legislation to many categories of health personnel and institutions.

Health Services for Agricultural Migratory Workers (1962). This act established a program of grants for family clinics and other health services for migrant workers.

Heart Disease, Cancer, and Stroke Amendments of 1965 (Regional Medical Programs). The purpose of this legislation was to "assist in combatting heart disease, cancer, stroke, and related diseases." Regional cooperative programs were established among medical schools, hospitals, and research institutions for programs of research, training, continuing education, and demonstrations of patient care in the fields of heart disease, cancer, stroke, and related diseases. The program was expanded under 1968 and 1970 amendments and by 1971 there were fifty-six regional medical programs covering all the states. However, with the passage of the National Health Planning and Resources Development Act of 1974, the regional medical programs were no longer funded as such and many of the programs were absorbed into the new health systems agencies.

*The Comprehensive Health Planning Amendments of 1966 ("Partnership for Health"). This legislation was designed to give the states more flexibility in the use of their grants-in-aid for public health work (through a block grant) and to encourage comprehensive health planning; it was the base for the state and areawide comprehensive health planning "A" and "B" agencies.

Communicable Disease Control Amendments of 1970. This legislation re-established the categorical grant program for control of communicable diseases, including tuberculosis, venereal disease, rubella, measles, Rh disease, poliomyelitis, diphtheria, tetanus, and whooping cough.

Family Planning Services and Population Research Act of 1970. This established an Office of Population Affairs under the Assistant Secretary for Health and Scientific Affairs. It added Title X, *Population Research and Voluntary Family Planning Programs*, to the Public Health Service Act. This authorized project, formula, training, and research grants and contracts for family planning programs and services (abortion excepted).

Emergency Health Personnel Act of 1970. This act authorized the Secretary to assign commissioned officers and other health personnel of the Public Health Service to areas designated as in critical need of health manpower. It provided the statutory base for the National Health Service Corps.

The National Sickle Cell Anemia Control Act and the National Cooley's Anemia Control Act (1972). These acts authorized grants and contracts for screening, and treatment, counseling, information and educational programs, and research related to these diseases. PL 94–278, 1976, broadened the program to include Tay–Sach's and other diseases (Title IX, *Genetic Diseases*).

Health Programs Extension Act of 1973. This act extended a number of programs whose authorizations were due to expire. These included migrant health, comprehensive health planning, Hill–Burton, allied health manpower training, regional medical programs, and family planning programs as well as programs under the Community Mental Health Centers Act and the Developmental Disabilities Services and Facilities Construction Act. (This is an example of a number of such acts that are periodically required to continue various grant programs. They may also, variably, include program revisions or additions.)

Emergency Medical Services Systems Act of 1973. This added a new title to the Public Health Service Act: Title XII—*Emergency Medical Services Systems.* It established a program of grants and contracts for the development and improvement of area emergency medical services systems, and for related research and training.

*The Health Maintenance Organization Act of 1973. This established a program of financial assistance for the development of health maintenance organizations.

Sudden Infant Death Syndrome Act of 1974. Part C, *Sudden Infant Death Syndrome*, was added to Title XI; this provides for public and professional informational programs related to this syndrome.

*National Health Planning and Resources Development Act of 1974. This consolidated and greatly revised the Hill–Burton, regional medical programs, and comprehensive health planning legislation.

Public Health Service Act Amendments (1975). This omnibus act extended and revised a number of health programs and activities: comprehensive public health services (Special Health Revenue Sharing Act of 1975); family planning (Family Planning and Population Research Act of 1975); migrant health; community health centers; National Health Service Corps and nurse training (Nurse Training Act of 1975). A separate grant program for community health centers was established under a new section of Title III (Section 330). Part D, *Hemophilia Programs* was added to Title XI, providing for projects for the development of diagnostic and treatment centers and blood component separation centers.

National Consumer Health Information and Health Promotion Act of 1976. The Public Health Service Act was amended by the addition of Title XVII—*Health Information and Promotion.* A program of grants and contracts was authorized for research and community programs related to health information, health promotion, preventive health services, and education in the appropriate use of health care. An Office of Health Information and Health Promotion was to be established in the Office of the Assistant Secretary for Health.

Omnibus Budget Reconciliation Act of 1981.   This legislation incorporated extensive budget reductions and program revisions. Included were changes in many grant programs funded under the Public Health Service Act. Many programs were extended with reduced funding. Some were otherwise limited, terminated, or underwent substantial changes. Particularly notable were the consolidation of a number of categorical programs into three block grants to the states. These were for *preventive health services*, combining eight programs for rodent control, water fluoridation, health education/risk reduction, home health agencies, public health services (formerly Section 314d), hypertension, emergency medical services, and rape crisis centers; *health services*, combining mental health, alcohol abuse and drug abuse programs; and *primary care* (community health centers). The legislation also provided for closing or transfer of the remaining Public Health Service hospitals and eliminated the entitlement of merchant seamen to care by the Public Health Service. A new program of grants related to the problem of adolescent pregnancy was established (a new Title XX—*Adolescent Family Life Demonstration Projects*).

HOSPITAL SURVEY AND CONSTRUCTION ACT OF 1946 ("HILL-BURTON ACT")

An Act to amend the Public Health Service Act to authorize grants to the States for surveying their hospital and public health centers and for planning construction of additional facilities, and to authorize grants to assist in such construction.

This act established the first of many post-World War II federally aided health programs.

Background

There was relatively little hospital construction during the years of the Great Depression and World War II. In 1944 a Commission on Hospital Care was organized by the American Hospital Association and the Public Health Service to study the national need for hospital facilities. The principles developed by the Commission and the Public Health Service are reflected in the Survey and Construction Act, introduced by Senators Hill and Burton, which became Title VI of the Public Health Service Act. The general language of this act is representative of legislation authorizing grants-in-aid to the states.

Summary of Major Provisions

- Grants to assist the states to *inventory* their existing hospitals and health centers and to *survey* the need and develop programs for the construction of such facilities.

- Grants to the states for *construction projects.*

- Federal funds for surveys and planning to be allotted to the states on the *basis of population.* Within its allotments, a state may receive a grant equal to 33-1/3 percent of these expenses.

  Funds for construction to be allotted annually to the states in accordance with a *formula* based on population and per capita income; from this allotment, grants may be made covering 33-1/3 percent of the cost of construction projects.

- In order to receive funds, a state must (among other provisions):

  a. Designate a *single state agency* to administer or supervise administration of the program, and establish a *state advisory council* to consult with the state agency. The council is to include representatives of nongovernmental agencies and state agencies concerned with hospitals, and representatives of the *consumers* of hospital services.

  b. Submit a *state plan* for the construction of facilities based on the statewide survey of need and conforming to regulations prescribed by the Surgeon General.

  c. Provide for the designation of a State Advisory Council to consult with the state agency in carrying out the act's purposes.

- The Surgeon General shall develop regulations concerning:

  a. The number of general hospital beds required to provide adequate hospital services in a state and the general methods by which such beds would be distributed. (Total beds for any state not to exceed 4.5 per thousand population, except up to 5.5 beds per thousand in less populated states.)

  b. The number of tuberculosis, mental disease, and chronic disease hospital beds required, and their distribution.

  c. The number and distribution of public health centers.

  d. The general manner in which the state agency will determine priorities for projects within a state, with special consideration to be given to hospitals serving *rural communities.*

  e. General *standards* for construction and equipment for hospitals.

  f. Requirements that the state plan provide for adequate hospital facilities for state residents without discrimination and for persons unable to pay therefor.[50]

- Grants are to be available only to states who enact or have enacted legislation providing for minimum standards of maintenance and operation for hospitals receiving federal aid under this program.

- The Surgeon General is to consult with a *Federal Hospital Council* in administration of this title. The council shall consist of eight members (plus the Surgeon General), including four representatives of consumers of hospital services.

By 1949, all the states and territories had had state plans approved by the Surgeon General. In most instances, the state health department had been designated as the responsible agency for the administration of the program. Most states now had licensure laws, most of which were applicable to all hospitals, not just those eligible for federal aid.

---

50. This section has been the subject of important litigation, with regard to racial segregation (see 1964 amendments) and the issue of provision of health care to the poor. The latter provisions were not implemented for some years as regulations were not developed. This is an example of the practical importance of rulemaking.

Amendments

The Hill-Burton Act has been amended frequently since its original enactment.

The *Hospital Survey and Construction Amendments of 1949* extended the program, increased the authorized funds and provided that the federal share of the costs of construction projects could be as much as 66-2/3 percent, depending on the relative need and economic status of the area involved. Additionally, grants were authorized for *research and demonstrations* relating to the development, utilization, and coordination of hospital services and facilities.[51]

The *Medical Facilities Survey and Construction Act of 1954* authorized grants for surveys and for construction of *diagnostic and treatment* centers (including hospital outpatient departments), *chronic disease* hospitals, rehabilitation facilities, and nursing homes.

Chronic disease hospitals were already included in the existing program, as were the other types of facilities when part of a hospital. The purpose of the legislation was to encourage the construction of such facilities by specifically earmarking funds for them and by including them even if they are not part of a hospital.

The *Community Health Services and Facilities Act of 1961*, which dealt primarily with the question of improving out-of-hospital services for the aged and chronically ill, included several amendments to the Hill-Burton program. Funds for *nursing home* construction were increased and the hospital research and demonstration grant program was extended to other medical facilities.

The *Hospital and Medical Facilities Amendments of 1964* extended the program and authorized grants specifically earmarked for *modernization* of hospitals with more priority than before being given to urban areas.

A new category of long-term care facilities was created that combined the chronic disease hospitals and nursing home categories, and its funding authorization was increased.

---

51. However, no funds were actually appropriated under this authorization until 1956. This, a frequent occurrence, is an example of the practical difference between authorization and actual appropriation of funds.

Grants were authorized to the state agencies for up to 50 percent of the costs of comprehensive regional or local area plans for coordination of existing and planned health facilities. (Planning to be done by state agencies or by designated local public or nonprofit groups.)

Language was added requiring that "any facility or portion thereof to be constructed or modernized, [is] to be made available to all persons residing in the territorial area of the applicant." This replaced the previous "separate . . . if like quality" provisions.[52]

The *Medical Facilities Construction and Modernization Amendments of 1970* again extended the program and added new provisions for federal loans and loan guarantees for construction and modernization. A new program of project grants was established for emergency rooms, communications networks, and transportation systems.

The *National Health Planning and Resources Development Act of 1974* revised the Hill–Burton legislation and incorporated it in a new Title XVI.

Administration.   Health Resources Administration.

COMPREHENSIVE HEALTH PLANNING AND PUBLIC HEALTH SERVICE AMENDMENTS OF 1966 ("PARTNERSHIP FOR HEALTH")

An Act to amend the Public Health Service Act to promote and assist in the extension and improvement of comprehensive health planning and public health services, [and] to provide for a more effective use of available Federal funds for such planning and services . . .

Background

In the years since the passage of the Public Health Service Act of 1944 the program of grants to the states for public health work had been expended largely by designating funds for specific purposes. As

52. A federal court had ruled (1963) this clause unconstitutional (Moses H. Cone Memorial Hospital *versus* Simkins); the Supreme Court refused (1964) to review this decision, thus in effect barring racial segregation in hospitals receiving federal funds under the Hill–Burton program.

of 1966, most of the federal support to the states for public health services was made available through one or another of such "categorical grants."[53] This system had come under considerable criticism as being excessively rigid, denying the state health department freedom to determine the allocation of these funds to public health problems. This legislation represented a departure from this approach to funding of public health services; it authorized "block" grants for public health programs and included provisions for the development of state and local planning for health services.

These amendments essentially involved a complete revision of Section 314 (Title III), which now referred to grants for *Comprehensive Health Planning* and for *Comprehensive Public Health Services.*

Summary of Major Provisions

Section 314a. Grants to the States for Comprehensive State Health Planning. In order to qualify for these funds, a state is to submit a "plan for comprehensive state health planning." This plan must designate a state agency (new or existing) to be responsible for the state's health planning functions, and provide for the establishment of a *state health planning* council to advise this agency. The council is to include representatives of state and local agencies, nongovernmental organizations and groups, and consumers of health services; a majority of the membership are to be representatives of consumers.

Section 314b. Project Grants for Areawide Health Planning. Grants are authorized to public or nonprofit organizations "for developing comprehensive regional, metropolitan area or other local area plans for coordination of existing and planned health services."[54]

Section 314c. Project Grants for Training, Studies, and Demonstrations. Grants to agencies, institutions, or other organizations for projects for training, studies, and demonstrations relating to the

---

53. Among these were cancer, chronic illness, dental disease, heart disease, mental illness, tuberculosis, and venereal disease.

54. The state planning agency became known as the "A" agency; and the substate agency, the "B" or "areawide" agency (or, "314a" and "314b" agencies).

development of improved or more effective comprehensive health planning.

Section 314d. Grants for Comprehensive Public Health Services. Grants to "assist the states in establishing and maintaining adequate public health services, including the training of personnel for state and local health work." Again, to qualify for these funds state plans for the provision of public health services are required and these plans are to be developed in accordance with the plan for comprehensive health planning. The federal share for public health programs under this section is to be 33-1/3 to 66-2/3 percent, and at least 15 percent of a state's allotment is to be used for mental health services.

Section 314e. Project Grants for Health Services Development. Grants are authorized to public or nonprofit private agencies, institutions, or organizations to cover part of the cost of:

- Providing services to meet health needs of limited geographic scope or of specialized regional or national significance;
- Stimulating and supporting, for an initial period, new programs of health services;
- Undertaking studies, demonstrations, or training designed to develop new or improved methods of providing health services.

Comprehensive Health Planning Amendments

The *Partnership for Health Amendments of 1967* extended the program and made several additions and modifications including:

- State plans for comprehensive health planning are to provide for assisting each health institution to develop a program for capital expenditures consistent with meeting the needs of the state for facilities and services most economically, efficiently, and without duplication.
- Representation of the *interests of local government* in areawide planning agencies is required.

- Section 314e was revised to transfer authority for studies and demonstrations to another section, and to limit the training provisions.[55]

The *Public Health Service Amendments of 1970* extended the program for an additional three years and made several further modifications including:

- State and areawide plans must include *home health services.*
- Areawide health planning councils are to be established to include representatives of the interests of local government, of the regional medical programs, and of *consumers* of health services. A majority of the members of such councils are to be representatives of consumers.

The *National Health Planning and Resources Development Act of 1974* completely revised the comprehensive health planning program as Title XV—*National Health Planning and Development.*

HEALTH MANPOWER LEGISLATION

The first federal legislation particularly addressed to the question of health manpower, except for certain temporary wartime programs, was the *Health Amendments Act of 1956.* This law authorized under Title III of the Public Health Service Act traineeships for professional public health personnel and for advanced training of professional nurses. A third provision amended the Vocational Education Act of 1946 specifically to authorize grants for programs for practical nurse training.

A program of formula grants to *schools of public health* was established in 1958 (PL 85–544). In 1960 there was added (PL 86–720) a program of project grants to schools of public health and schools of nursing or engineering providing graduate or specialized public health training. The *Graduate Public Health Training Amendments of 1964* broadened eligibility for project grants to include other institutions providing such training.

---

55. Subsequently, a number of community health centers were developed under this section. In 1975, with the establishment of a new separate program for these centers, Section 314e was repealed.

A large body of health manpower legislation has since developed. The following are brief summaries of the major statutes.

Health Professions Education Assistance Act of 1963

This act inaugurated, under Title VII of the Public Health Service Act, the program of *construction grants* for teaching facilities: grants for the construction or rehabilitation of facilities for training of physicians, dentists, pharmacists, podiatrists, nurses,[56] or professional public health personnel, these contigent on increased first year enrollments. Also authorized was a program of *student loan funds* at schools of medicine, osteopathy, and dentistry.[57]

Nurse Training Act of 1964

This act added Title VIII, *Nurse Training* to the Public Health Service Act. This authorized separate funding for construction grants for schools of nursing and extended eligibility to associate degree programs and diploma schools; these were also contingent on increased enrollment. Also authorized were project grants to the schools to improve and expand their training programs, and formula grants to diploma schools. Provision was also made for the establishment of *student loan funds* at schools of nursing.

Health Professions Educational Assistance Amendments of 1965

These amendments authorized a program of grants to "improve the quality of schools of medicine, dentistry, osteopathy, optometry and podiatry." These were *basic improvement* (institutional) grants related to enrollment and contingent on increased enrollment, and *special improvement* grants. *Scholarship* grants were also authorized for these schools, plus schools of pharmacy. The student loan program was expanded, with provisions for partial cancellation for phy-

56. In schools with baccalaureate or graduate degree programs.

57. Following the general pattern of loan funds established under the National Defense Education Act of 1958. Students of optometry and veterinary medicine were subsequently included (PL 88-654, 89-709).

sicians, dentists, and optometrists practicing in shortage areas, and eligibility was extended to students of pharmacy and podiatry.

Allied Health Professions Personnel Training Act of 1966

This act established programs of *construction* and *improvement grants* for training centers for allied health professions,[58] generally patterned after those in the previous legislation. *Advanced traineeships* for allied health professions personnel were authorized, as were project grants related to the training of new types of health technologists. Other provisions included additional loan cancellation for physicians, dentists, and optometrists practicing in poor rural areas and revolving funds for student loan funds under Titles VII and VIII.

Health Manpower Act of 1968

This act extended, with some changes, most of the previous programs. Among the changes were the extension of the institutional and special project grants to schools of pharmacy and veterinary medicine and the addition of students of veterinary medicine to the scholarship program. These schools had become eligible for construction grants in 1966 (PL 89-709).

Health Training Improvement Act of 1970

This act provided for institutional grants for new schools of health professions and extended, with some changes, the grant programs for allied health professions. Authorization was added for *special project* grants and contracts related to training or retraining of allied health personnel. Also authorized was a program of grants and contracts for projects related to encouraging and assisting the entry into allied health professions training of individuals of financial, educational, or cultural need, and provision was made for grants for *scholarships, work-study programs*, and *student loan funds.*

58. Defined as institutions that provide "education leading to a baccalaureate or associate degree or a higher degree in medical technology, dental hygiene, or other curriculums specified by regulations. . . . "

Comprehensive Health Manpower Training Act of 1971

This act comprised extensive and complex amendments. It extended the program of construction grants for health research and teaching facilities, raised the latter grant ceiling to 70 to 80 percent, and mandated an opportunity for review and comment by the appropriate 314a and 314b agencies. Provisions for construction loan guarantees and interest subsidies were added.

The previous institutional grants were replaced by a new system of *capitation grants* for each student enrolled in health professional schools, again contingent upon increased first-year enrollment and upon submission of plans for projects for improvement of teaching programs in at least three of nine specified categories.[59] *Start up* assistance to new schools of medicine, osteopathy, and dentistry was authorized, also in the form of capitation grants.

Special project grants and contracts were authorized for a wide variety of activities related to professional education in priority areas and the utilization of health personnel. Additionally, grants were authorized to schools in *financial distress*.

A new program of grants and contracts, *health manpower education initiative awards*, was authorized for health and educational entities to support a wide variety of projects for the purpose of "improving the distribution, supply, quality, utilization, and efficiency of health personnel and the health services delivery system"; these awards are to be coordinated with the area's regional medical program. Additional grants were authorized for special projects related to enrollment of students who might be expected to practice in shortage areas, and students who are financially or otherwise disadvantaged.

The *loan* provisions were broadened to provide up to 85 percent cancellation for health professionals practicing for three years in shortage areas. *Scholarships* for needy students were increased and provision was made for the total amounts available for the scholar-

---

59. These covered such activities as curriculum improvements (including shortening), interdisciplinary training, training for new roles or types of personnel (including physician assistants and nurse practitioners), teaching of health care organization; training in clinical pharmacology, nutrition, and management of drug and alcohol abuse, programs related to admission and retention of disadvantaged students, and projects related to training primary care health professionals and family medicine.

ship funds to be increased according to numbers of students enrolled from low income backgrounds. A new *physician shortage area* scholarship program was established for medical students who agree to practice primary care (one year for each scholarship year) in an area of physician shortage or with substantial number of migrant agricultural workers.

Another new program included grants for training, traineeships, and fellowships in family medicine; annual capitation grants for approved graduate training programs for physicians and dentists in primary care and other designated shortage areas of care; grants for advanced training, traineeships, and fellowships for health professions teaching personnel; and grants related to the use of computer technology in health care.

Finally, there were a number of miscellaneous provisions relating to health manpower. A National Health Manpower Clearinghouse was established. The Secretary was directed to use his best efforts to provide, to each county certified to be without the services of a physician, at least one physician in the National Health Service Corps. The Comptroller General was directed to conduct a study of *health facilities construction costs.* The Secretary was directed to arrange for a study (preferably by the National Academy of Sciences) of the annual per student *educational cost* of schools of health professions (including nursing) and to prepare a report on the parts of Title VII related to health professionals education. A number of studies related to health manpower was mandated.

Nurse Training Act of 1971

This act extended the construction grant program, increased the grant ceiling to 67 to 75 percent of costs, and added provisions for loan construction guarantees and interest subsidies. The program of special project grants was broadened to cover a wide variety of activities related to nursing and interdisciplinary training; contract authorization was added, and provision was made for grants to schools in *financial distress.*

The program of formula grants to diploma schools[60] was replaced by annual *capitation* grants for nursing schools, generally contingent

---

60. This is an example of a program that was not actually funded and thus was never implemented.

on increased enrollment, with additional amounts authorized for further enrollment increase, and for schools with training programs for nurse midwives, family health nurses, and other nurse practitioners. An additional requirement for these grants was that a school submit a plan to carry out projects in at least three of several categories related to improved nursing training. A separate program of *start up* grants was authorized for new nurse training programs.

The advanced traineeships and the student loan program were continued, with provision made for loan cancellation of up to 85 percent after five years of full-time nursing employment, and, for practice in an area of shortage, of up to 85 percent after three years. *Half-time* students were also made eligible for loans. The *scholarship* program was extended and expanded, with half-time students becoming eligible.

Additionally, grants and contracts were authorized to health or educational entities for activities related to the enrollment in schools of nursing of persons such as veterans with health field experience, the financially and otherwise disadvantaged, and licensed practical nurses. Finally, the Secretary was directed to report to Congress on the administration and impact of the Title VIII programs.

Nurse Training Act of 1975

This act extended and revised the various programs related to nursing education and in addition made new grant and contract authorization for special projects including advanced nursing training and nurse practioner programs, and cooperative arrangements (including) mergers) among hospital training programs and academic institutions. (Amendments in 1979 again extending these programs allowed the authority for financial distress grants for schools to expire and added a program for traineeships for nurse anesthetists.)

Health Professions Educational Assistance Act of 1976

The program of *capitation grants* to professional schools was extended and provisions for grants to schools of public health were added. Conditions include maintenance of previous levels of first-year enrollment, and requirements that medical schools have up to 50 percent (by 1980) of their residency programs in primary care (internal medicine, family medicine, or pediatrics) and reserve positions in their third-year classes for U.S. students enrolled in foreign medical schools.[61] The program of *construction grants* for teaching facilities was continued with new authorization for grants for construction of primary care teaching facilities for physicians and dentists. The authority for research facility construction grants was repealed. New authorization for *special projects* included grants (or contracts) for departments of family medicine, area health education center programs, programs related to the transfer of U.S. students from foreign medical schools, training programs for physicians' assistants and dental auxiliaries, residency programs in general medicine or pediatrics, occupational health training and education centers, family medicine training, and programs related to recruitment and admissions of disadvantaged students. There was also broadened authorization for *start-up grants* for new schools, grants for schools in financial distress, for cooperative interdisciplinary training, and for a wide variety (twenty-one) of other projects and programs.

Also authorized were special project grants for *schools of public health* and *graduate programs in health administration* for the development or expansion of programs in biostatistics and epidemiology; health administration, health planning or health policy analysis and planning; environmental or occupational health; or dietetics and nutrition. *Institutional* grants were authorized (excluding schools of public health) to support graduate programs in health administration, hospital administration, and health planning.

A number of programs (some of which had not in fact been funded) for scholarships, loans, and traineeships were repealed or phased out. The major program for professional *student loans* was continued with some modifications and certain limitations. (For example, interest rates were raised from 3 percent to 7 percent and the ability to discharge loan obligations via bankruptcy was restricted.) Provisions were made for loan forgiveness, related to service in the National Health Service Corps or practice in a manpower shortage area. Scholarships for exceptionally needy first year students were authorized.

---

61. Provisions subsequently modified.

A new program of *traineeships* for students in schools of public health[62] and in graduate programs in health administration was established. The National Health Service Corps program was revised and extended, including the procedure for designation of health manpower shortage areas and the assignment of National Health Service Corps personnel.

A number of restrictions were placed on the entrance to the United States of foreign physicians as immigrants or exchange visitors. For example, such physicians must have passed Parts I and II of the examination of the National Board of Medical Examiners (or an equivalent examination).

Health Manpower Amendments (1981)[63]

Among the many provisions of these amendments were revisions of the National Health Service Corps (NHSC) program, including reduction in the number of new NHSC scholarships to be offered, and provisions designed to encourage the use of the placement option of private practice in health manpower shortage areas. Re-evaluation of the criteria for designation of health manpower shortage areas was required. Grants were authorized to schools of medicine and osteopathy for improvement of departments of family medicine (in addition to the establishment and maintenance of such departments) and priority is given to support of family medicine residency programs. A new program was established for the support of preventive medicine residency training. The requirement for maintenance of increased student enrollment as a condition of grants for educational institutions was eliminated. The program of capitation grants for schools of nursing was allowed to expire; financial distress grants were added. Priority for nurse practioner traineeships is to be given to students in nurse–midwifery.

Administration.   Health Resources Administration.

62. Schools of public health were for the first time brought under the grant programs of the Title VII comprehensive manpower legislation. Previously, the schools have been provided for under separate project and institutional grant and traineeships provisions in Title III.

63. Title XXVII, Omnibus Budget Reconciliation Act of 1981.

Note

The health manpower legislation is a good example of the categorical grant programs and their incremental development. Also, it should be kept in mind that the awarding of grants is subject to criteria and priorities set forth in the legislation and in regulations and that not all programs authorized are actually funded by appropriations.

HEALTH MAINTENANCE ORGANIZATION ACT OF 1973

An Act to amend the Public Health Service Act to provide assistance and encouragement for the establishment and expansion of health maintenance organizations, and for other purposes.

A new title, XIII, *Health Maintenance Organizations*, is added to the Public Health Service Act.

Summary of Major Provisions

Financial Assistance for the Development of Health Maintenance Organizations

A program of financial assistance was established for the development or expansion of health maintenance organizations. This comprised:

- Grants and contracts to determine the feasibility of development or expansion of individual health maintenance organizations;
- Grants and contracts for planning projects;
- Grants, contracts, and loan guarantees for initial development;
- Loans and loan guarantees for initial operating costs (to offset, when necessary, losses during the first thirty-six months).

Basic medical services are to be provided for a set, periodic payment fixed under a community rating system. These services are:

- Physician services
- Inpatient and outpatient services

- Medically necessary emergency health services
- Short-term outpatient evaluative and crisis intervention mental health services (not over twenty visits)
- Medical treatment and referral services for alcohol and drug abuse
- Laboratory and x-ray services
- Home health services
- Preventive services (including voluntary family planning and infertility services, and preventive dental care and eye examination for children)

Nominal additional payments may be required for specific basic services.

The basic health services payment may be supplemented by nominal charges for specific services (copayment) unless this is determined to be an undue barrier to the delivery of health services.

Supplemental health services are to be made available to enrolled members who wish to contract for them. These are:

- Intermediate- and long-term care
- Vision care and dental and mental health services not included under basic services
- Provision of prescription drugs

At least 20 percent of the appropriated funds are to be allocated to rural health maintenance organizations.

Professional services that are provided as basic services are, in general, to be provided through health professionals who are members of the staff of the health maintenance organizations or through medical groups or individual practice associations.

The requirements for a health maintenance organization include:

- Evidence of fiscal responsibility
- Enrollment of persons broadly representative of the age, social, and income groups within the area served; except that not more than 75 percent of the members may be enrolled from a medically underserved population, unless the area served is a rural area
- A policymaking board, at least one-third of whose membership are (enrolled) members of the organization, and with equitable representation of the medically underserved population

- Arrangements for a quality assurance program
- Provision of medical social services and health education services
- Provision for continuing education for its health professional staff

Organizations serving Medicare and Medicaid beneficiaries are not required to provide basic services that are not compensated under these programs, nor to fix payments by community rating.

Employees Health Benefit Plans

Every employer of twenty-five or more persons is to include in health benefit plans offered to employees the option to enroll in health maintenance organizations that are providing services in the areas in which the employees reside.

Restrictive State Laws and Practices

State requirements that prevent an entity from functioning as a health maintenance organization shall not apply. Specifically, pre-empted restrictions are:

- Requirement of approval by a medical society of services furnished
- Requirement that physicians constitute all or a percentage of the governing body
- Requirement that all or a percentage of physicians be permitted to participate in the provision of services
- Certain requirements for insurers
- Prohibition of solicitation of members through advertising of services, charges, or other nonprofessional aspects of an organization's operation

Quality Assurance

A new part is added to Title III of the Public Health Service Act: Part K—*Quality Assurance*. Provision is made to conduct research and evaluation programs respecting the effectiveness, administration, and enforcement of quality assurance programs.

Amendments

The *Health Maintenance Organization Act Amendments of 1976* included provisions designed to make the requirements under the Act somewhat less stringent. A health maintenance organization (HMO) could, at its option, offer any of the supplemental health services as part of its basic health benefits. Preventive dental care for children was omitted from the required preventive services and immunizations, well-child care from birth and periodic health evaluations for adults were added to these services. The offering of supplemental services was made optional. Services (within specified limits) could be provided by individual practitioners by contract with the HMO. (Health professionals providing such services need not be members of groups or practice associations.) Requirements for open enrollment were retained, with modifications, only for larger and well-established HMOs. Existing HMOs were given four years to establish community rating systems. An additional provision required that HMOs receiving reimbursement from Medicare or Medicaid must be federally qualified.

The *Health Maintenance Organization Amendments of 1978* extended and made numerous revisions and adjustments to the program. Additions included a new program of loans and loan guarantees for acquisition of ambulatory care facilities and for related equipment, a program for training HMO administrators, medical directors, and other managerial personnel, and provisions for technical assistance for HMO development.

The *Health Maintenance Organization Amendments of 1981*[64] included provisions to permit increased flexibility in the organizational arrangements of HMOs, particularly in the area of physicians' services. The "community rating" requirements are modified with the establishment of an optional "community rating by class" system whereby differential premiums could be set; classes (e.g., certain age groups) can be derived by actuarial or other means that predict differences in use of HMO services. Additional provisions reflect continuing concern with the fiscal integrity of health maintenance organizations.

---

64. Title IX, Subtitle F, Omnibus Budget Reconciliation Act of 1981.

Administration.   Office of Health Maintenance Organizations.

NATIONAL HEALTH PLANNING AND RESOURCES DEVELOPMENT ACT OF 1974

An Act to amend the Public Health Service Act to assure the development of a national health policy and of effective state and area health planning and resource development programs, and for other purposes.

Two new titles, XV and XVI, were added to the Public Health Service Act. They superseded and greatly modified the previous programs established under Sections 314a and 314b of Title III (Comprehensive Health Planning), Title VI (Hill–Burton), and Title IX (Regional Medical Programs). A brief summary of the major provisions follows.

Title XV. National Health Planning and Development

National Guidelines for Health Planning

The Secretary is to issue *national health policy planning* guidelines, formulated in consideration of stated *national health priorities.* A National Advisory Council on Health Planning and Development is established.

Health Systems Agencies

Provision is made for the establishment of *health service areas* and *health systems agencies* (HSAs) throughout the United States.

A health service area, to be designated by the state governor, will in general have a population of 500,000 to 3,000,000, and have boundaries coordinated with those of Professional Standards Review Organizations and existing planning areas. Except under certain circumstances, each standard metropolitan statistical area is to be within the boundaries of one health service area.

A nonprofit (health planning or development) corporation, public regional planning body, or unit of local government may apply for designation as a health systems agency. Each agency is to have a governing body of which a majority are to be area residents and consumers.

The stated purposes of the agencies are: 1) improving the health of area residents; 2) increasing the accessibility, acceptability, continuity, and quality of health services; and 3) restraining costs and preventing duplication of health services.

The functions of the agencies include the collection and analysis of data, establishment of *health systems plans* (HSPs) and *annual implementation plans* (AIPs), and the making of grants and contracts from an Area Health Services Development Fund to be established. They are to review and approve or disapprove the use of federal funds in the area for health services or resources development; and periodically review all institutional health services for appropriateness; and annually recommend to the state agency projects for modernization, construction, and conversion of medical facilities.

Planning grants will be made annually to each health service agency according to a per capita formula. The basic grant is to be the lesser of $0.50 per person in the area or $3,750,000.

State Health Planning and Development

The Secretary is to enter into agreements with the governors of each state for the designation of a *state health planning and development agency* (SHPDA). If such an agreement is not in effect after four years, no funds may be made available under the Public Health Service Act, Community Mental Health Centers Act or the Comprehensive Alcoholic Abuse and Alcoholism Act for the development or support of health resources in the states. A Statewide Health Coordinating Council is also to be established.

The functions of the state agency are to: 1) conduct health planning for the state; 2) prepare (from the HSPs) and annually review a state health plan for submission to the Coordinating Council; 3) assist the council in review of the state medical facilities plan (see Title XVI) and other functions; 4) administer a *state certificate of need program*; 5) periodically review all institutional services in the state with regard to appropriateness.

The State Health Coordinating Council is to be appointed by the governor, with a majority of the members to be appointed from among nominees from the health systems agencies.

The Council is to: 1) annually review and coordinate the HSPs and AIPs; 2) review annually the state health plan; 3) annually review the budgets of the health systems agencies; 4) review grant applications for federal funds under the Public Health Service Act, Community

Mental Health Centers Act, or the Comprehensive Alcohol Abuse and Alcoholism Act. Disapprovals may be reviewed, at state request, by the Secretary.

Grants are to be made to the state agencies for up to 75 percent of their costs.

Grants may be made to (not more than six) state agencies for the purpose of demonstrating their effectiveness in regulating rates for the provision of health care.

A *national health planning* information center is to be established to support the health planning and resource development programs.

The Secretary is to develop uniform systems for calculating services costs, volumes, and rates to be charged, for cost accounting and for classifying health services institutions.

The Secretary is to assist by grants or contracts the development of *centers for health planning.*

Title XVI. Health Resources Development

Purpose, State Plan, and Project Approval

The purpose of this title is to provide assistance for projects for modernization of medical facilities, construction of new outpatient facilities, construction of new inpatient facilities in areas of recent rapid population growth, and conversion of facilities for the provision of new health services, and for projects related to the elimination of safety hazards and the avoidance of noncompliance with licensure or accreditation standards.

A *state medical facilities plan* must be submitted by the state agency. The plan must, among other requirements, be approved by the Statewide Health Coordinating Council as consistent with the state health plan.

Project applications must, among other requirements, include reasonable assurances that the assisted facility will be made available to all persons in the area and that a reasonable volume of services will be made available to persons unable to pay therefor. Each application is to be reviewed by the appropriate health systems agencies.

Allotments

Allotments are to be made to the states from appropriated funds on the basis of population, financial need, and need for medical facilities.

Requirements include the stipulation that not more than 20 percent of a state's allotment may be obligated for construction of new inpatient facilities and not less than 25 percent is to be obligated for outpatient facilities for medically underserved populations, including rural populations.

Loans and Loan Guarantees

Provision is made for a program of loans and loan guarantees for projects approved under Part A (Purpose, State Plan, and Project Approval).

Project Grants

Provision is made for construction or modernization projects designed to eliminate or prevent safety hazards or to avoid noncompliance with state or voluntary licensure or accreditation standards. Such grants are to be made only to public or quasi-public entities.

General Provisions

General provisions related to judicial review of project disapprovals, recovery of funds, financial statements, definitions, and technical assistance.

The *federal share* of the costs of a grant-assisted project may be up to 66-2/3 percent (up to 100 percent in the case of an urban or rural poverty area).

Amendments

The *Health Planning and Resources Amendments of 1979* made a number of revisions and additions to the health planning program. Provisions were added addressing the fostering of competition. A general outline was set forth of the process to be used in selecting members of governing bodies and subarea councils of the health systems agencies, a majority to be consumers of health care services and broadly representative of the area residents. The definition of "provider" of health care services for purposes of HSA membership was modified. There were provisions addressing the need for the integration of mental health and alcoholism and drug abuse resources in the health system plans. The *certificate of need* provisions were revised to include "major medical equipment that will be used to provide services to hospital inpatients."[65] Health maintenance organizations were exempted from the certificate of need requirements relating to inhospital facilities and services.

The *resources development* (Hill–Burton) provisions were also revised. The allotment (formula) grants to the states for facilities construction were eliminated.[66] The loan and loan guarantee provisions were restricted to purposes of the *discontinuance and conversion* of unneeded hospital facilities and services, the construction of new outpatient facilities, and the construction of inpatient facilities in areas of rapid population growth. Project grants were authorized, largely for public hospitals, for elimination of safety hazards, or meeting accreditation standards. Project grants were also authorized for construction of outpatient facilities apart from hospitals and for conversion of unneeded facilities to outpatient or long-term care use. A new program was also established to provide grants and technical assistance for hospitals to encourage discontinuance of inpatient hospital facilities and services, or their appropriate conversion. Grants were authorized to the state health planning and development agencies for activities related to reduction of excess hospital capacity.

Health planning amendments in 1980 (PL 96–538) made technical amendments to the program and added a provision that a certificate of need need not be required for acquisition of major medical equipment for institutional health services, or capital expenditures related solely to research purposes. Health planning amendments in 1981[67] (PL 97–35) provided for reduced levels of funding for health systems agencies, for termination or area consolidation in the case of HSAs whose funding is deemed inadequate to support an effective HSA, and allows HSAs to accept contributions from health insurance companies (similar to previous provisions for major employers). State governors may request the elimination of federal designation and funding of HSAs in their states, with all health planning functions then to be carried out by the State Health Planning and Development agencies and the Statewide Health Coordinating Councils. The time limit for state compliance with certificate of need requirements was

---

65. This provision was designed to prevent the circumvention of the certificate of need laws by the acquisition of CT Scanners by, for example, physicians, with arrangements for their use by hospital inpatients.

66. The original major feature of the Hill–Burton program thus came to a close.

67. Title IX, Subtitle E, Omnibus Budget Reconciliation Act of 1981.

extended. There are also provisions for waiver, for any or all HSAs, of the requirement for conducting appropriations review, review of proposed use of federal funds, and the collection and publication of data on hospital costs.

Administration. Health Resources Administration.

MENTAL RETARDATION FACILITIES AND COMMUNITY MENTAL HEALTH CENTERS CONSTRUCTION ACT OF 1963

> An Act to provide assistance in combating mental retardation through grants for construction of research centers and grants for facilities for the mentally retarded and assistance in improving mental health through grants for construction of community mental health centers, and for other purposes.

Congressional interest in the problem of mental health was first expressed in the *Mental Health Act of 1946*, which specifically provided for the inclusion of mental health problems in the grant-in-aid programs of the Public Health Service Act and established the National Institute of Mental Health patterned after the National Cancer Institute. The *Mental Health Study Act of 1955* authorized grants to facilitate a program of research into resources and methods for care of the mentally ill,[68] and in 1956 the *Health Amendments Act* added special project grants particularly directed to the problems of state mental hospitals. Legislation addressed to the problem of mental retardation was added in 1963 in the *Maternal and Child Health and Mental Retardation Planning Amendments.*

Summary of Major Provisions

Construction of Research Centers and Facilities for the Mentally Retarded — "Mental Retardation Facilities Construction Act"

- Amends Title VII of the Public Health Service Act to authorize grants to assist in the construction of facilities for research relating to mental retardation. Federal participation: up to 75 percent.

---

68. The resultant Joint Commission on Mental Illness and Health published a final report, *Action for Mental Health*, in 1961.

- Grants for the construction of university-affiliated facilities providing a full range of inpatient and outpatient services; for demonstrating specialized services for the mentally retarded; or for clinical training of physicians and other specialized personnel. Federal participation: up to 75 percent.

- Grants to the states for the construction of community facilities for the mentally retarded; patterned after the Hill–Burton program. Federal share: 33-1/3 to 66-2/3 percent.

Construction of Community Mental Health Centers— "Community Mental Health Centers Act"

Grants to the states for construction of community mental health centers, also generally patterned after the Hill–Burton Program. Federal share: 33-1/3 to 66-2/3 percent.

Training of Teachers of Mentally Retarded and Other Handicapped Children

Extends and strengthens existing programs for training teachers of mentally retarded and deaf children,[69] and expands them to include the training of teachers of other handicapped children.

Amendments to the Mental Retardation and Community Mental Health Centers Legislation

The 1965 amendments to this legislation included provisions for grants to assist in meeting the initial cost of professional and technical personnel for community mental health centers (30 to 75 percent), and grants to institutions of higher education for construction of facilities for research in the field of education of handicapped children.

The *Mental Health Amendments of 1967* extended the program of grants for construction and initial staffing of community mental health centers and amended the term "construction" to include acquisition of existing buildings. The *Mental Retardation Amend-*

---

69. Legislation (PL 85-929, 1958) authorizing grants to educational institutions and agencies for training teachers of mentally retarded children.

ments of 1967 extended the program of construction grants for university-affiliated and community facilities for the mentally retarded, and established a program of initial staffing grants analogous to those for community mental health centers. A new program authorized grants to educational institutions for the training of physical educators and recreation personnel for mentally retarded and other handicapped children and for related research and demonstration projects.

The *Alcholic and Narcotic Addict Rehabilitation Amendments of 1968* added new provisions to the Community Mental Health Centers Act, relating to alcoholism and narcotic addiction: grants for construction and initial staffing of facilities for the treatment and rehabilitation of alcoholics[70] and narcotic addicts and grants for special training programs and evaluation studies relating to narcotic addiction services.

The *Community Mental Health Centers Amendments of 1970* extended the program of construction grants and changed the definition of construction to include the acquisition of land. The duration of initial staffing grants was lengthened to eight years and, for centers in poverty areas, the grant ceiling was increased to 70 to 90 percent. Provision was also made for centers in poverty areas to begin operation (for eighteen months) without furnishing all the required services of a community mental health center.[71] Additionally, grants were authorized to local agencies for development of community mental health services in rural or urban poverty areas.

The program of grants for facilities and services for alcoholics and narcotic addicts was also extended,[72] the duration of the staffing grants lengthened, and the grant ceiling increased, for centers in poverty areas. Special project grants were authorized for training, surveys, treatment, and rehabilitation projects.

---

70. These facilities to be associated with other mental health services program, including community mental health centers.

71. Services required for federally funded centers were:

"1. Inpatient services
2. Outpatient services
3. Partial hospitalization services—must include at least day care services
4. Emergency services provided 24 hours per day . . .
5. Consultation and education services [for] community agencies and professional personnel."

72. The alcoholism section of this program had not yet been implemented.

The Community Mental Health Centers Act was further amended by the addition of a part of the mental health of children. This authorized grants for construction of facilities[73] for the mental health of children, the cost of professional and technical personnel for new facilities or new services, and for training and program evaluation.

The *Comprehensive Drug Abuse Prevention and Control Act of 1970*[74] included provisions broadening the scope of narcotic addiction programs to include drug abuse and drug dependence, authorized grants for programs and activities related to drug education and special project grants for drug abuse and addiction treatment and rehabilitation.

The *Comprehensive Alcohol Abuse and Alcoholism Prevention, Treatment and Rehabilitation Act of 1970* provided a new separate statutory base for programs directed to alcohol abuse and alcoholism, as did the *Special Drug Action Office and Treatment Act* of 1972 for programs directed to drug abuse.

The *Developmental Disabilities Services and Facilities Construction Amendments of 1970* extended the mental retardation programs and broadened the language of the legislation to include other neurological handicapping conditions. The *Developmentally Disabled Assistance and Bill of Rights Act* (1975) provided a new separate statutory base for programs for mental retardation and other developmental disabilities.

The *Community Mental Health Centers Amendments of 1975* extended and revised the community mental health centers program. The required services were increased to twelve, including programs of specialized services for children and the elderly, and there were provisions for governing bodies or advisory committees made up of area residents.

The *Mental Health Systems Act of 1980* extensively revised the community mental health program, including provisions for comprehensive state mental health systems. This legislation was however largely superseded by the *block grants* to the states for mental health

---

73. Associated with a community mental health center or other appropriate facility.

74. Title II of this legislation is the *Controlled Substances Act*. It contains provisions for drug abuse related control and enforcement by the Department of Justice.

and alcohol and drug abuse that were established by the *Omnibus Budget Reconciliation Act of 1981.*

ECONOMIC OPPORTUNITY ACT OF 1964 ("ANTIPOVERTY PROGRAM")

An Act to mobilize the human and financial resources of the Nation to combat poverty in the United States.

Summary of Major Provisions

Work Training and Work Study Programs

- Establishes the Job Corps (conservation camps and residential training centers).
- Work-training programs for unemployed youths and young adults (Neighborhood Youth Corps).
- Work-study programs in colleges and universities for students from low income families.

Urban and Rural Community Action Programs

- Grants for antipoverty programs to be planned and carried out at the community level. Programs are to be administered by the communities and are to mobilize all available resources and facilities in a coordinated attack on poverty.
- Grants to the states for basic adult education programs.
- Voluntary assistance program for needy children (information and coordination office).

Antipoverty Programs in Rural Areas

- Loans to low income rural families.
- Assistance for housing, sanitation, education, and child care programs for migrant farm workers.
- Indemnity payments to farmers for pesticide-contaminated milk.

Assistance to Small Business Concerns

Loans and management training for small businesses.

Work Experience Programs

Grants for experimental and demonstration work experience and training programs for unemployed persons on public assistance.

Administration and Coordination

Establishes the Office of Economic Opportunity and provides for administration of the act. Authorizes the program *Volunteers in Service to America* (VISTA).

Exemption of Income for Public Assistance Purposes

Exemption of part or all of earnings under the Economic Opportunity Act from consideration as income or resources of public assistance recipients.

Office of Economic Opportunity (Executive Office of the President)

- Direct responsibility for the *Job Corps, community action programs, VISTA*, and the programs for migrant farm workers;
- Indirect (delegated) responsibility for the work study, adult education, and work experience programs (Department of Health, Education and Welfare); the work training programs (Department of Labor); the special rural programs (Department of Agriculture); and the small business programs (Small Business Administration);
- Coordination of the poverty-related programs of all federal agencies.

Community Action Programs

The legislation defines a community action program eligible for federal assistance as one that:

> Mobilizes and utilizes resources, public or private . . . in an attack on poverty; provides services, assistance and other activities [which] give promise

of progress toward the elimination of poverty or a cause or causes of poverty . . . ; is developed, conducted and administered with the *maximum feasible participation of residents of the areas and members of the groups served;* and is conducted, administered or coordinated by a public or nonprofit agency, or combination thereof.

Community action programs could be conducted in such fields as employment, job training and counseling, health, vocational rehabilitation, housing, home management, welfare, and special remedial and other noncurricular educational assistance.

Among the many programs that were developed under the community action provisions, and that were given statutory recognition in amendments to this title, were the Office of Economic Opportunity (OEO) neighborhood health centers, the Head Start child development programs, the legal services programs and family planning and drug rehabilitation programs.

The Economic Opportunity Act, often controversial, was much amended, and many administrative changes were made. The VISTA program was combined with the Peace Corps in a new ACTION agency, the Head Start program was placed in the Department of Health, Education and Welfare's Office of Child Development, and the neighborhood health centers were transferred to the Public Health Service. A nonprofit *Legal Services Corporation* for the legal assistance programs was established by the Legal Services Corporation Act of 1974.

In 1975, under the *Headstart, Economic Opportunity and Community Partnership Act*, the Office of Economic Opportunity was abolished and replaced by the independent *Community Services Administration*, which administered the community action programs until it was in turn abolished in 1981. (Some of the programs are being continued under state community services block grants.)

FEDERAL FOOD, DRUG AND COSMETIC ACT

The Act of 1906, popularly known as the *Pure Food and Drug Act* or the "Wiley Act"[75] defined adulterated and misbranded foods and drugs[76] and prohibited them from interstate commerce. Its passage

75. For Harvey W. Wiley, Chief of the Department of Agriculture's Bureau of Chemistry, who campaigned for this legislation.

76. "Adulteration" is defined as a departure from prescribed standards of strength, quality, or purity.

followed several years of crusading by reformers and journalists concerning unwholesome and adulterated foods and the widespread use of patent medicines. Among subsequent amendments were those to include standards for quality of canned foods (1930) and to provide for voluntary inspection of sea food packing establishments (1934).

Federal Food, Drug and Cosmetic Act of 1938

This act was an extensive new law that replaced the original legislation, greatly expanding its provisions relating to food and drugs and adding provisions for regulation of medical devices and cosmetics. It was passed after much controversy and only after the deaths of ninety people from a contaminated elixir of sulfanilamide overcame the opposition. The legislation provided that no new drug could be marketed before the submission of a *new drug application* (NDA) to be accepted only when accompanied by the manufacturer's proof of safety.[77] This act has been frequently amended. The following are particularly important statutes.

Food Additives Amendment of 1958

The purpose of this legislation was to prohibit the use of food additives that have not been adequately tested for safety. Among the provisions directed to assuring the safety of additives was the "Delaney Clause" (named for Representative James Delaney who sponsored it), which stated that "no additive shall be deemed to be safe if it is found to induce cancer when injested by man or animal, or if it is found, after tests which are appropriate for the evaluation of the safety of food additives, to induce cancer in man or animal" (e.g., laboratory animals). This clause was invoked to limit the sale of the artificial sweeteners cyclamate and saccharine and has become quite controversial.[78]

77. Previously, action could only be taken by the seizure and proscription of already marketed drugs.

78. Much of the controversy relates to the stringent application of test results in laboratory animals mandated by the clause.

Drug Amendments of 1962
("Kefaufer-Harris Amendments")

These amendments were finally passed following widespread publicity about the adverse effect of thalidomide. They made extensive revisions strengthening the provisions related to the regulation of therapeutic drugs. Among these was the requirement that new drug applications (NDAs) must include reports of investigations showing that the drug proposed for marketing is *effective* as well as safe. Previously approved new drug applications (i.e., for drugs marketed before the enactment of this statute) may be withdrawn if there is a "lack of substantial evidence that the drug will have the effect it is represented to have."

Medical Devices Amendments of 1976

These amendments, providing for strengthening the regulation of medical devices,[79] were passed, after the failure of previous bills, in the setting of increasing reports of adverse effects of medical devices (for example, complications from the Dalcon Shield intrauterine device).

Three classifications of devices were established (to be determined for each case by *classification panels*):

Class I. Devices for which *general* (regulatory) *controls* including those related to registration, records and reporting, and good manufacturing practices are sufficient to provide reasonable assurance of safety and effectiveness.

Class II. Devices that are determined to require *performance standards* to provide such assurance.

Class III. Devices that require *premarket approval.* This class is for devices that are to be used in supporting or sustaining life, that are of substantial importance in preventing impairment of health, or that present a considerable risk of illness or injury. (Examples of Class III devices are cardiac pacemakers and artificial

---

79. "Devices" include instruments, apparatus, machines, implants, and other articles (including components, parts, and accessories) intended for use in diagnosis, treatment, or prevention of disease or to affect the structure or any function of the body.

heart values.) Applications for premarket approval are to include full reports of all investigations of the safety and effectiveness of the device. Provision is made for investigational use of devices.

Administration

This legislation is administered by the Food and Drug Administration.

A NOTE TO THE READER

Many details of the book will be altered by changing events. This is particularly true of these sections dealing with federal legislation and the organization of federal agencies.

In the case of congressional activity this problem can be dealt with without undue difficulty if the interested reader will, once having acquired a basic understanding of the progression of the laws, develop a systematic approach to keeping abreast of developments. One method would be the regular scanning of the *Congressional Quarterly* or the *U.S. Code Congressional and Administrative News.* Systematic review of one of the many Washington newsletters would also be useful. Examples of these are the *Washington Report on Medicine and Health* and the letters published by the various interested associations, such as the American Public Health Association, the American Public Welfare Association, and the Association of American Medical Colleges. A regular *Memorandum* published by the Special Committee on Aging, United States Senate, is good for matters affecting the elderly, including Social Security amendments.

With regard to the activities and reorganizations of the executive agencies, the above newsletters are helpful and direct inquiries to the agency of interest will elicit information, although the substantive quality varies widely. Some put out regular newsletters. Significant reorganizations and all administrative regulations are published in the *Federal Register.* Those who are involved with federal programs usually take care to watch for these.

Much useful information about programs and issues can be found in congressional committee reports and hearings related to specific legislation.

Obtaining Documents

Single copies of bills, laws, committee hearings, and reports can usually be obtained from the House or Senate Document Room, Washington, D.C.; zip codes 20515 and 20510, respectively. (Enclose a self-addressed label.) These can often also be obtained from the congressional committees or from the offices of individual senators and representatives. Similarly, single copies of many reports and publications can be obtained from the relevant agencies. The U.S. Government Printing Office publishes a monthly catalog of published documents, which are for sale at usually reasonable prices.

SELECTED READINGS

The first three books illustrate well the workings of the legislative process:

The Dance of Legislation, Eric Redman (New York: Simon and Schuster, 1973).

Politics, Science and Dread Disease, Stephen P. Strickland (Cambridge, Massachusetts: Harvard University Press, 1972).

A Sacred Trust, Richard Harris (New York: New America Library, 1966). History of the Medicare legislation.

The Development of the Social Security Act: A Memorandum on the History of the Committee on Economic Security and Drafting and Legislative History of the Social Security Act, Edwin E. Witte (Madison: University of Wisconsin Press, 1963).

Social Security Programs in the United States, U.S. Department of Health, Education and Welfare, Social Security Administration. This is an excellent summary of programs related to the Social Security Act. It is revised periodically, following major amendments.

Politics of Federal Grants, George E. Hale and Marian L. Palley (Washington, D.C.: Congressional Quarterly Press, 1981).

Welfare Medicine in America: A Case Study of Medicaid, Robert Stevens and Rosemary Stevens (New York: The Free Press, 1974).

Information Sources

How Our Laws Are Made, Charles I. Zinn (House of Representative Document No. 93–377, 1974).

Guide to the Congress, 2nd edition (Washington, D.C.: Congressional Quarterly, 1979).

Congressional Directory. Published for each session of Congress by the United States Government Printing Office.

Congress and Health. Published for each Congress by the National Health Council. An excellent summary of the Congress and the legislative process including Congressional committees and their jurisdictions.

Congressional Quarterly and Almanac (Washington, D.C.: Congressional Quarterly, Inc.). Weekly summary and commentary on congressional activities.

U.S. Code Congressional and Administrative News (St. Paul, Minnesota: West Publishing Co.). Monthly congressional summary with texts of newly passed laws and related committee reports.

Washington Report on Medicine and Health (Washington, D.C.: McGraw-Hill, Inc.). A weekly commentary on federal events, particularly legislative.

1981 Medicare Explained (Chicago, Illinois: Commerce Clearing House Inc., 1981).

NOTE: There are many official *government document depositories*, containing selected documents, in public and university libraries throughout the country. Some of these are *regional depositories* which receive copies of most documents published by the Government Printing Office.

7 THE ROLE OF STATE AND LOCAL GOVERNMENTS

In principle, the responsibility for the general health, safety, and welfare of the people resides with the states, which enact and implement appropriate laws under the inherent police powers of the sovereign state. Despite the steadily rising influence of the federal government in recent years, these basic powers and responsibilities have remained with the states, which have a major and expanding role in many aspects of health care, including extensive regulation of health facilities and manpower. Certain powers and functions are delegated to the local governments of counties, cities, and towns either directly or through the state charters, which permit many cities and towns to function with considerable autonomy.

THE SPECTRUM OF STATE AND LOCAL HEALTH FUNCTIONS

Health-related activities and services and their organization vary greatly from state to state in accordance with their financial means and priorities. They include traditional public health activities, many personal health services, educational programs, and a variety of regulatory functions.

Public Health Activities

Historically, the prime role of the states and localities in health has been related to sanitation, communicable disease control, and the assurance of the quality of water and food supplies. These, together with the collection of vital statistics have comprised traditional "public health" activities to which have more recently been added water fluoridation, control of air pollution and radiation, and the regulation of disposal of hazardous chemical wastes. These functions are important to the health of the community as a whole and require the exercise of organized governmental responsibility.

Personal Health and Medical Care Services

Personal health and medical care services provided by the states and localities include:

- *Institutional services* for long-term conditions such as tuberculosis and other chronic diseases, mental illness, and mental retardation. Most of these services are beyond the capacity of the private sector or local communities and are typically provided by the states. Many counties and municipalities operate short-term general hospitals, particularly for care of the poor. Long-term care institutions, including nursing homes, are also operated by many local jurisdictions, usually counties.

- *Ambulatory services* for communicable disease control (e.g., venereal disease, tuberculosis, and immunization clinics), plus a variety of services related to disease prevention and health promotion such as maternal and child health, school health, nutrition, family planning, dental, chronic disease (e.g., diabetes and hypertension screening), alcohol and drug abuse treatment, and health education. Additionally, many therapeutic services are provided through outpatient departments, health centers, and home care programs.

Regulation of Institutions, Organizations, and Occupations

Many types of health institutions and organizations are licensed and monitored by the states. Hospitals and nursing homes are most widely regulated, but organizations such as pharmacies, clinical laboratories, blood banks, and ambulance services are regulated in many states. Health and safety codes are established and monitored for housing, institutions, and industry. In response to the rise in health care costs, many states have developed programs directed to cost control such as "certificate of need" (for construction of facilities) and rate setting (see Chapter 10).

Health insurance companies are regulated under insurance laws; Blue Cross–Blue Shield, and in some instances, health maintenance organizations, under specific enabling legislation. Some states require that certain minimum benefits be included in health insurance contracts, and some mandate that special benefits such as treatment for mental illness, and alcohol and drug abuse be included or available. (A few states, notably Rhode Island, have developed their own insurance plans for catastrophic illness.) Workmen's compensation insurance programs for job-related injury and illness are mandated. A number of states now regulate the manufacture and dispensing of drugs, particularly those subject to abuse.

Many health professions and occupations are licensed by the states (see Chapter 4). Under the licensure laws these health personnel come under varying degrees of ongoing regulation. For example, many states now require participation in continuing education programs as a condition for physicians' continued licensure.

Other Regulatory Activities

The states carry out health planning functions through a federally supported system of local health system agencies (HSAs), state health planning and development agencies (SHPDAs), and state health coordinating councils (SHCCs). These systems are variably integrated with other state regulatory activities such as the certificate of need programs.

Other activities by some states include laws related to the control of drugs subject to abuse, and the control of drug costs by encouraging prescribing by generic name and restricting drugs that will be paid for under Medicaid; laws mandating automobile seat restraints for children; laws delineating patients' rights in hospitals and nursing homes; and many others. Some states are very active in regulation, others are much less so.

Education and Training

There are many programs for health manpower education and training in the state colleges, universities, and other institutions. These include schools of medicine, nursing, dentistry, and many others. Local schools and colleges, including community colleges, provide educational programs for many types of health personnel. Additionally, some states are supporting specific aspects of health manpower education, particularly physician education, in areas of perceived need such as family practice departments (mandated for some state medical schools) and family practice residency training programs.

Federal–State Programs

About 30 percent of the funds for health programs in the states comes from the federal government, mostly in the form of grants-in-aid. (See Chapter 6.) These funds may supplement existing state activities or be designed to encourage the states to expand or institute new programs deemed of importance by the federal government. They have greatly influenced the organization and scope of state health programs, beginning with the passage of the Hill–Burton Hospital Survey and Construction Act in 1946, which spurred state activities in health planning and hospital licensure in addition to health facilities construction. Funding includes general block grants and categorical grants, including those for the health planning agencies; community mental health, communicable disease control, emergency medical systems, lead paint poisoning prevention, maternal and infant care, and children and youth projects; vocational rehabilitation and other programs for the mentally and physically handicapped; and Medicaid. Under new federal legislation[1] many categorical grants are being combined into health block grants with fewer

---

1. The Omnibus Budget Reconciliation Act of 1981.

federal requirements (but fewer total funds, a point of some contention by the states).

The federal government also contracts with the states for the surveying and certification of hospitals and nursing homes for Medicare participation.

Health-related services in the states, and as delegated to the counties, cities, and towns, are provided by a complex and everchanging variety of agencies and organizations in patterns that differ from state to state. At the state level, many of them are lodged in *departments of public health* but others are typically lodged in other departments. For example, there is often a separate state department of mental health; licensing of health manpower may be a responsibility of departments of education; vocational rehabilitation programs are often administered by separate agencies;[2] occupational health (industrial hygiene) is usually lodged in state departments of labor; and school health is commonly the responsibility of boards of education. Recently, several states have placed environmental control programs in separate agencies.

STATE HEALTH DEPARTMENTS

In most of the states, primary responsibility for traditional public health services and a varying number of other health-related services are lodged in a separate *state department of health*. There is also usually a *state board of health* (sometimes called public health council), with varying advisory, policy, and administrative functions, with members generally appointed by the governor, often with legislative consent. (In a few states state professional societies participate in the approval process.)[3] The majority of members of state boards of health are professionals, most frequently physicians and dentists. In over half the states there is some consumer representation. The chief executive officer (health officer, director, commissioner) is also usually appointed by the governor or by the board. In some states, the health agency is combined with one or more other agencies, most

2. In many states, for example, services for the blind are administered separately by separate agencies, such as *Commissions for the Blind*.

3. See Daniel J. Gossert and C. Arden Miller, "State Boards of Health, Their Members and Commitments," *American Journal of Public Health* 63, no. 6 (June 1973:486–493.

often the department of public welfare (now commonly termed department of social services).

State departments of health delegate many functions to the local departments, providing them general liaison, consultation, and special services as needed, a notable exception being major regulatory activities.

Figure 7–1 shows the organization of a state health department.

In 1978, the state of Michigan enacted a widely commented upon model public health code after many months of joint discussions and hearings by a legislative council and governor's commission. The act recodified the many previously existing public health laws and consolidated most health-related activities in a reorganized state department of health. It included explicit provisions for the strengthening of local health units and programs and reflected current regulatory priorities, including a restructuring of the system of occupational licensure.

Association. The *Association of State and Territorial Health Officials* (ASTHO) addresses the interests of state health agencies. Among other activities, the organization publishes an annual inventory of the agencies' expenditures, which is a useful source of data about state health programs.[4]

LOCAL HEALTH DEPARTMENTS

The traditional "basic six"[5] functions of local public health agencies are:

1. Collection of *vital statistics* of births, deaths, and reportable diseases.

2. Control of communicable diseases, including tuberculosis and venereal diseases.

3. Environmental sanitation, including water quality and supervision of foods and eating places.

---

4. See Association of State and Territorial Health Officials, *Inventory of Programs and Expenditures of State and Territorial Health Agencies, Fiscal Year 1978*, (The National Public Health Program Reporting System, 1980).

5. As set forth in the report *Local Health Units for the Nation* by Haven Emerson (The Commonwealth Fund, 1945).

Figure 7–1. A State Department of Public Health.

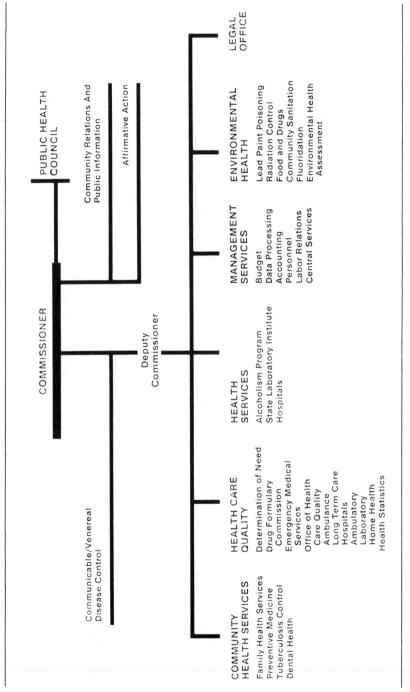

4. Public health laboratory services.

5. Maternal and child health, including school health.

6. Health education.

Many other activities have been added in recent years but these remain central functions of most local health departments.

With a few exceptions, mostly in some rural western counties,[6] all areas of the United States are served by local health units—county, city, town, or, in a few instances, combined city and county. Where there is no local health unit, services are provided by regional or district offices of the state health department. The number and scope of services provided vary greatly.

There are usually local *boards of health* with members appointed by elected officials—county commissioners or supervisors, mayors, or town selectmen. The *health officer* is typically appointed by the board generally in accordance with qualifications set by the state. Generally, though not invariably, the health officer is a physician; many are part time. The relationship between state and local health agencies varies greatly among the states.[7]

Staff of a local health unit will include as a minimum the health officer, one or more public health nurses, and one or more sanitary engineers or sanitarians. With increasing scope of responsibilities, the number and types of professional and technical staff will increase commensurately and may include dentists, social workers, health educators, nutritionists, epidemiologists, statisticians, special laboratory personnel, and many others.

Where many and complex services are provided, the health officer serves as director or commissioner of an organized department of health with appropriate divisions; here the basic unit for provision of direct services to the population is usually the district *health center*. Large health departments may be partially decentralized, with district health officers.

The health center houses services such as maternity and family planning clinics, well baby and child health clinics, tuberculosis and

6. But also in parts of New York State and all of Delaware, Rhode Island, South Dakota, and Vermont.

7. See Gordon De Friese, et al., "The Program Implications of Administrative Relationships between Local Health Departments and State and Local Government," *American Journal of Public Health* 71, no. 10 (October 1981): 1109–1115.

venereal disease units, dental clinics (usually for children), nutrition and health education services, and field personnel for environmental health programs. Some health centers in low income communities have in recent years been providing treatment as well as preventive services for children, usually in cooperation with a local hospital.

Many local health departments have also sponsored and established, often in cooperation with community groups, a variety of *community health centers* in both urban and rural areas. Many have also established home health agencies, usually by expansion of their public health nursing units or existing home care programs.

Some counties and large cities operate general hospitals. These systems are in some instances combined with local health agencies in *departments of health and hospitals* (examples are Boston and Denver).

STATE DEPARTMENTS OF MENTAL HEALTH

There is generally a separate mental health department, sometimes called the *department of mental hygiene.* The director (commissioner), usually a psychiatrist, is appointed by the governor according to legislatively established qualifications. In the past, the major responsibility of these departments has been the operation of large hospitals for the mentally ill and institutions for the mentally retarded. However, with the trend toward community mental health and deinstitutionalization, they manage an increasingly complex system of after-care programs, community mental health centers, halfway houses, and community residences. Programs for treatment of alcohol and drug abuse are also important activities of these departments.

There may be some decentralization of state mental health activities to regional and local levels but to a lesser degree than with local health units. There have been some experimental programs for the integration of health and mental health services at the local level (e.g., Florida and Massachusetts).

STATE MEDICAID AGENCIES

Medicaid accounts for a third or more of many state health expenditures. The Medicaid program is usually administered by the state department of public welfare, although in about ten instances this responsibility has been lodged in the health department. The Medicaid agencies establish individual eligibility for the Medicaid program and are responsible for the payment of providers of services and for general standard setting and monitoring. The federal government establishes guidelines and regulations and pays 50 to 83 percent of the costs of the program.

All states except Arizona now participate in Medicaid. The coverage of federally aided public assistance recipients (AFDC) and supplemental security income (SSI) recipients is federally mandated. The states have the option of including other welfare recipients and the medically indigent; about half do so.

These units also administer the federally mandated health screening program for Medicaid eligible children, *Early and Periodic Screening, Diagnosis and Treatment* (EPSDT), which generally contracts with a variety of local ambulatory facilities and private physicians for evaluation and treatment of these children.

UMBRELLA AGENCIES

In recent years a number of state and local jurisdictions have attempted to consolidate and streamline health and social welfare services by combining related departments and agencies into one overall administrative structure. These "umbrella agencies" or "super agencies" have involved varying combinations of departments of health, hospitals, mental health, public welfare, rehabilitation, youth services, and others. Examples of such amalgamations are the North Carolina Department of Human Resources, the Massachusetts Executive Office of Human Services, and the Suffolk County (New York) Department of Health Services. Many of these agencies have been politically controversial. An example is the New York City Health Services Administration, which was established in 1967 and dismantled in 1977.

SELECTED READINGS

"Community Health and the Law," George A. McKray, *Public Health Reports* 79 (1964): 654.

Public Health Administration and Practice, 7th edition, John J. Hanlon, and George E. Pickett (St. Louis: The C.V. Mosby Company, 1979).

"Role of State and Local Governments in Relation to Personal Health Services," Sagar C. Jain, ed., *American Journal of Public Health* 71 (1981): Supplement.

8 VOLUNTARY AGENCIES AND ORGANIZATIONS

There is a wide variety of nonprofit organizations that are supported in whole or in part by private contributions and whose activities are directed to specific or general health or social welfare problems. They have been termed *voluntary agencies.* In a broad sense, the term could refer to any nonprofit organization, including hospitals, as distinct from public ("official") and for-profit (proprietary) entities. The term as used here excludes institutions.

Typically, voluntary agencies have been developed by private citizen groups, and have predominantly lay boards and a variable mix of professional and volunteer staff. They are considered legally as "charitable and educational institutions" under Internal Revenue Service regulations (for tax exemption purposes).

Many are national bodies concerned with specific diseases or problems, with local chapters and affiliates. Examples are the American Cancer Society, the American Heart Association, the National Kidney Foundation, the American Lung Association,[1] and the National Association for Mental Health. The activities of such organizations are in general public education and the financial support of studies, research, and often training in areas of their special concern. Some

---

1. This is the oldest voluntary health agency, with origins in the Anti–Tuberculosis Society of Philadelphia (1892) and the National Association for the Study and Prevention of Tuberculosis (1904), later known as the National Tuberculosis and Respiratory Disease Association and recently renamed the American Lung Association.

also provide specific services; for example, the Planned Parenthood Federation operates over 700 family planning clinics and the American Cancer Society provides many cancer patients services such as sick room supplies and equipment, and transportation for treatment.

Other agencies are community based and usually organized primarily for provision of direct services. Examples are visiting nurse associations; family service agencies that provide counseling and other social services; and a wide variety of referral and counseling programs devoted to a myriad of problems, from drug abuse to suicide prevention.

Many organizations have evolved into standard components of the health care system (such as visiting nurse associations), and the social welfare system (such as family service agencies).

The American Red Cross is unique in being a quasi-official agency, chartered by Congress. It serves as the designated U.S. agency in national and international disaster relief, serves members of the armed forces, and operates a nationwide system for volunteer blood donation and distribution.

There are also many coordinating councils and agencies in which a number of voluntay organizations are loosely joined for planning, coordination, mutual education and interests, or fund-raising purposes. Among these are local community councils, united funds and community chests (many of these functioning as part of the United Way of America). One of the largest such local organizations is the Federation of Jewish philanthropies of New York, which raises and distributes funds to 130 affiliated agencies including hospitals, family services, community centers, and homes for the aged. Nationally, the National Health Council comprises 84 organizations, including some federal agencies.

SELF-HELP (MUTUAL AID) ASSOCIATIONS

These organizations further mutual support, education, and group advocacy for persons who share certain illnesses or problems. Examples are Alcoholics Anonymous, United Ostomy Association (ileostomy and colostomy surgery), and Mended Hearts (heart surgery). Some are closely coordinated with related national organizations (such as Reach to Recovery, for women who have undergone breast surgery, now a program of the American Cancer Society); others remain independent of established organizations and professionals (such as Alcoholics Anonymous). Parents of handicapped children have been particularly active in the formation of such mutual aid and advocacy groups.

PROFESSIONAL ASSOCIATIONS

Often considered under the rubric of voluntary agencies are the many associations formed by professionals, agencies, and institutions to further their mutual interests and professional goals. They are also known as *membership associations.* Some consider these "trade associations" but most have to a greater or lesser degree activities directed toward general health problems and issues. Examples are the American Medical Association, American Nurses' Association, American Hospital Association, American Public Health Association, and the Association of American Medical Colleges. Many have large budgets, are active lobbyists, and support a wide range of activities. Some have large state and local counterparts or affiliates such as state and county medical societies. Most professional associations, however, are much smaller and more informal, focusing on specialties or subspecialties (American Association of Public Health Dentists), scientific and research areas (American Society for Clinical Investigation, American Association for the Study of Liver Diseases) and techniques (Association for the Advancement of Medical Instrumentation).

PHILANTHROPIC FOUNDATIONS

Foundations have generally been established by single donors or families, and they aid a wide variety of activities primarily through the making of grants. They often fund relatively large research and demonstration projects, educational facilities and programs, and new services and programs. Foundations nationally active in the health field include the Robert Wood Johnson Foundation, W.K. Kellogg Foundation, the Kresge Foundation, the Henry J. Kaiser Family Foundation, and the Rockefeller Foundation. Most have areas of special interest, such as ambulatory care programs and personnel (Robert Wood Johnson Foundation), education (Carnegie Foundation for the Advancement of Teaching), and building construction and renovation (Kresge Foundation). Some are active solely in the health field (Kaiser Family Foundation); others have more general purposes (Rockefeller Foundation). Some limit their activities to a geographical area (Cleveland Foundation).

Some foundations have had important impact. Examples are the Carnegie Foundation's support of Abraham Flexner's survey of medical schools (reported in 1910) and the Rockefeller philanthropies' support of a hookworm central program in the southern states (through the Rockefeller Sanitary Commission, established for that purpose in 1909) and support of full-time medical school clinical professorships, notably at Johns Hopkins University Medical School (through the General Education Board in 1914), a system that became a model for other medical schools.

In 1970, foundations came under federal regulation (the Tax Reform Act of 1969). Now, for example, in order to qualify for tax exemption, a foundation must expend annually all of its investment income, or 5 percent of its assets.

PUBLIC INTEREST GROUPS

These organizations grew out of the consumer activism movement of the 1960s. They are primarily directed toward advocacy, studies, and research in areas of wide consumer interest and public policy. An example in the health field is the Health Research Group, part of the Ralph Nader organization Public Citizen, which has been particularly active in the areas of occupational health and safety and drug and product safety.

SELECTED READINGS

Voluntary Health and Welfare Agencies in the United States, Robert H. Hamlin, New York: Schoolmaster's Press, 1961, p. 309–318.

"Voluntary Health Agencies." In John J. Hanlon and George E. Pickett, *Public Health Administration and Practice*, 7th edition (Saint Louis: The C.V. Mosby Company, 1979).

Directories

Encyclopedia of Associations, 15th edition, Denise S. Akey, ed. Detroit: Gale Research Company, 1980. An extensive listing of national organizations, agencies, and associations. Regularly updated.

The Foundation Directory, 7th edition, Marianna O. Lewis, ed. New York: The Foundation Center, 1979.

9 PHARMACEUTICALS, CLINICAL LABORATORIES, BLOOD BANKS, AND MEDICAL EQUIPMENT, SUPPLIES, AND SERVICES

A multitude of items and services are required for the operation of the health care system. Most of these are supplied by a diverse collection of business firms and corporations that make up the *pharmaceutical industry*, the *medical equipment and supply industry*, and the *clinical laboratory system*. A specialized group of *blood banks*, nonprofit and proprietary, is another important complex of services. There is also a great variety of other special services including optical and dental laboratories, management consultants, hospital and nursing home management services, information and computer systems, food services, and laundry and maintenance services.

THE PHARMACEUTICAL INDUSTRY

A basic distinction is made between prescription drugs and nonprescription drugs. Prescription drugs are sold only by physician's prescription. Advertising about specific drugs is directed only to physicians. Because the manufacturers follow this self-imposed ban on advertising to the public, these are sometimes called *ethical drugs* and their manufacturers, the *ethical drug industry*. Nonprescription drugs (proprietary drugs, over-the-counter drugs, OTCs) are sold without prescription and advertising is directed to the public (e.g., Bayer aspirin).

A given drug may be known by three names:

- The *chemical name* uses the terminology that describes its chemical structure (e.g., 7–chloro–1, 3–dihydro–1–methyl–5–phenyl–2H–1, 4–benzodiazepin–2–one).

- The *generic name* is the established or official name for the drug (e.g., diazepam).

- The *brand name* (proprietary drug name) is the registered trademark given by its manufacturer (e.g., Valium, manufactured by Roche Products, Inc.).

Since 1964 the generic (nonproprietary) name of a new drug is assigned by the U.S. Adopted Names Council (USAN), which includes representatives of the American Medical Association, the U.S. Pharmacopeial Convention and the American Pharmaceutical Association, and the participation of the Food and Drug Administration.

Biologics. Biologics (biological products, biologicals) differ from drugs in that they are, or are derived from, living organisms and cannot be synthesized or readily standardized by chemical or physical means. They tend to be chemically less stable than drugs, their safety cannot be as easily assured, and they are never as chemically pure as drugs. Examples are vaccines, antitoxins, and blood plasma products.

Federal Regulation

Food and Drug Administration. The pharmaceutical industry is extensively regulated by the federal Food and Drug Administration (FDA) through the *Bureau of Drugs* and the *Bureau of Biologics.*

Since the passage of the 1938 Food, Drug and Cosmetic Act (which replaced the Pure Food and Drug Act of 1906) a New Drug Application (NDA) must be submitted and approved before a new drug can be marketed. This also must be done for each new use of a drug. Information required for an NDA includes a full report on investigations in animals and humans[1] to show that the drug is safe;

---

1. Under the 1962 amendments, an investigational new drug application (IND)—or, more precisely, a "Notice of Claimed Investigational Exemption for a New Drug"—must be filed to permit testing on human beings. This testing is then done in three phases: I) healthy

a full statement of the composition of the drug and the method of manufacture; and samples of labeling, including a detailed drug brochure (package insert). Under the 1962 amendments NDAs must also include demonstration of effectiveness as well as safety. About 2,500 prescription drugs that had been approved between 1939 and 1962 were therefore evaluated for effectiveness by National Academy of Sciences/National Research Council review panels. This led to the withdrawal of a number of these drugs (particularly combination drugs containing more than one ingredient) from the market. A separate review process has addressed over-the-counter drugs.

The FDA has, since 1938, determined whether a given drug could be sold over-the-counter or by prescription only. A number of formerly prescription drugs have recently been approved as OTCs. The FDA also regulates prescription drug advertising. Over-the-counter drug advertising is regulated by the Federal Trade Commission. The manufacturing plants for drugs and biologics are inspected periodically by the appropriate bureau.

Drug Enforcement Administration. This agency, a part of the Department of Justice, regulates narcotics and dangerous drugs, including the registration of all manufacturers, distributors, dispensers, and prescribers.

State Regulation

Antisubstitution Laws and Generic Prescribing. In the 1950s nearly all states passed laws that forbade pharmacists to substitute nonproprietary (generic) equivalents for prescribed brand name drugs. These statutes were said to prevent the dispensing of counterfeit drugs. In the 1970s most of these laws were repealed or modified and at present virtually all states permit, and in some cases require, substitution of generic for brand name drugs under specified conditions. These are now often termed "drug product selection" laws and are considered cost-saving measures.

---

volunteers; II) small-scale patient studies; and III) wide-scale patient studies. If the drug is then judged suitable for marketing, an NDA will be filed. The entire process of filing an FDA review is long and complex and has led to considerable controversy about a possibly inappropriate delay in new drug approvals ("drug lag").

Licensing and Registration.   All states license pharmacies and pharmacists. Many also register pharmacists and physicians for the purpose of controlling dangerous and narcotic drugs, including such requirements as special record keeping and certain prescribing and dispensing restrictions.

The Structure of the Pharmaceutical Industry

There are about 800 prescription drug companies in the United States. (They may also make or distribute over-the-counter drugs.[2]) Of these, 100 or so account for 95 percent of all prescription drugs sold and have most of the research and development capacity. Drug companies may be independent (including those formed by merging two or more companies) or divisions or subsidiaries of large diversified corporations. Some of the largest of the companies (based on dollar sales volume) are listed in Table 9-1. Table 9-2 shows the application of the drug manufacturers' revenue dollar.

New drugs are patentable. A *patent* is a legal monopoly granted by the federal government for a period of seventeen years from the time it is issued.[3] A patent can cover new chemical entities, and new ways of making them, but not drug dosage forms. A company with a patented drug may license other companies to make and sell this drug in exchange for payment (royalties). The patent is designed as a method for encouraging research and new ideas by allowing inventors to "capture" the profits from their inventions.

The central importance of research for new drugs results in large research expenditures. The information and research necessary to process an NDA through the FDA is large and costly. Approval by the FDA begins a marketing campaign that includes advertising to physicians in various forms, including visits to doctors by *drug detail men*, who inform them of this new product.

If there is no patent, other companies may make and sell the drug either under their own brand name or under the generic name. Drugs for sale by generic names are often sold at a substantially lower price. The critics of the industry argue that the difference results in vast profits from brand name drugs. The defenders of the industry argue

---

2. Several thousand firms make or distribute OTCs.

3. The useful life of a drug patient may be shortened by up to several years by the required FDA approval process.

Table 9-1.   Dollar Sales, Major Drug Companies (*$ millions*).

Roche Laboratories	700
Wyeth Laboratories	700
Merck, Sharpe and Dahme Division	600
U.S. Pharmaceutical Company (Squibb)	600
Pfizer Pharmaceuticals	536
Lederle Laboratories	506
Lilly Pharmaceutical Division	475
Smith Kline & French Laboratories	411
Searle Pharmaceuticals	386
Ayerst Laboratories	350
Upjohn Pharmaceutical Division	342
Abbott Pharmaceutical Products	340
A.H. Robins Company	307
Ciba-Geigy Pharmaceuticals	300
Ross Laboratories	250
Schering Corporation	250
Merrell-National Laboratories Division	235
Parke Davis & Company	208

Source: Adeline B. Hale and Arthur B. Hale, *The Medical and Healthcare Marketplace Guide.* (Miami: International Bio-Medical Information Service, Inc., 1978). This is a list of companies with sales over $200 million in 1977. Some of these companies sell products other than prescription drugs and these sales dollars are included here. All except A.H. Robins are corporate divisions or subsidiaries.

Table 9-2.   Where the Drug Manufacturer's Sales Dollar Goes (*percent*).

31.2	Cost of goods sold
20.0	Promotion (advertising)
15.5	Administration
12.0	Taxes
9.1	Profits
9.0	Research
2.5	Quality control
0.7	Medical school aid

Source: M. Silverman and P.R. Lee, *Pills, Profits and Politics* (Berkeley: University of California Press, 1974), pp. 28-29.

that behind the brand name stands the reputation of the company for high quality performance and the price differential reflects quality differences, as well as the cost of research and development.

Pharmacies. Prescription drugs may only be dispensed by licensed pharmacists (or physicians) who work in institutional (mainly hospital) or community pharmacies. According to the National Center for Health Statistics, in 1973 there were about 56,000 community pharmacies of which about 10,600 were *chain pharmacies* (four or more pharmacies under the same ownership). Examples of large chains are Rexall and CVS.

Associations

Pharmaceutical Manufacturers Association (PMA) — One hundred and forty-three of the larger drug companies.

American Pharmaceutical Association — The professional association for pharmacists.

National Association of Retail Druggists — Owners of independent drugstores and employed pharmacists.

Drug Compendia

The United States Pharmacopeia, 20th Revision / *The National Formulary*, 15th edition, (Rockwell, Maryland: U.S. Pharmacopeial Convention, Inc., 1979). These standard and somewhat overlapping compendia have been consolidated with the acquisition in 1975 of the National Formulary by the U.S. Pharmacopeial Convention. The now combined volume contains descriptive monographs for recognized drugs and pharmaceutic ingredients (by generic name), setting forth chemical and physical properties and standards for purity, assay, and storage.

Physicians' Desk Reference (PDR). Published annually by Medical Economics, Oradell, New Jersey. A compendium essentially of the official (FDA approved) drug company brochures. Supported by drug manufacturers and distributed to all physicians. This is the most widely used drug reference.

AMA Drug Evaluations, 4th Edition. AMA Department of Drugs, in cooperation with the American Society for Clinical Pharmacology and Therapeutics. (Chicago: American Medical Association, 1980). This is a discussion of drugs and their clinical uses.

CLINICAL LABORATORIES

Clinical (medical) laboratories carry out tests on blood and other body fluids and tissues for the detection, diagnosis, and monitoring of disease. They are located in hospitals, physicians' offices, and public health agencies or are independent, privately owned corporations.

Exclusive of physicians' offices, there are approximately 15,000 clinical laboratories, roughly divided between hospitals and independent labs.[4] In recent years, there has been a rapid growth of high-volume independent laboratories including corporate chains, encouraged by the development of automotatic analyzers for chemical testing. Many clinical labs are now owned by drug and chemical companies (such as Abbott, Dow, Smith Kline & French, and Upjohn). Examples of other large corporate laboratories are Damon, MetPath, and United Medical Laboratories.

The first automated analyzer was introduced by Technicon in 1957. It was followed in 1966 by the now widely used SMA 12/60 (Sequential Multiple Analyzer) that can process 60 blood samples, 12 tests each, per hour. More advanced, computerized systems have since been marketed by Technicon, Hyal, Dupont, and other companies.[5]

Laboratories are directed by physicians (usually pathologists) or other scientists (such as biochemists and microbiologists). Some are highly specialized for performance of certain complex testing ("reference laboratories") or for special purposes (public health laboratories). Many hospitals are sharing large central laboratories that permit high volume and diverse services.

Regulation

The Center for Disease Control regulates laboratories in interstate commerce by licensure, standards setting, and proficiency testing under the Clinical Laboratory Improvement Act of 1967. The FDA establishes standards for diagnostic reagents. About half the states license clinical laboratories and/or laboratory personnel. Some regulate the billing practices of independent laboratories and physician's office laboratories. The Joint Commission on Accreditation of Hospitals surveys hospital laboratories as a part of its hospital accreditation procedure.

4. "National Survey of Hospital and Non-Hospital Clinical Laboratories," *Laboratory Management* 17 (March 1979).

5. Technicon's SMAC (computerized) system introduced in 1974 can select twenty of twenty-four tests and process 150 samples (3,000 tests) per hour.

Associations

College of American Pathologists — Activities include voluntary accreditation of labs.

American Society of Clinical Pathologists — Clinical pathologists, clinical scientists, and medical technologists. It participates in the accreditation of schools and training programs for lab personnel and offers certification and proficiency testing.

American Society for Medical Technology — Clinical laboratory personnel.

American Clinical Laboratory Association — Large independent laboratories.

BLOOD BANKS

The American Association of Blood Banks defines a blood bank as a facility that recruits at least 100 donors per year and draws, processes, stores, and distributes human blood and its derivatives. Blood banks supply blood for use by hospitals. They include:

Hospital blood banks, which draw and process blood primarily for their own needs.

Community blood banks, which are nonprofit centers supplying local area hospitals.

The American Red Cross, which includes fifty-nine regional centers, with mobile units.

Commercial blood banks, which are for-profit centers using paid donors only.

There are about 5,000 blood banks, of which the majority are in hospitals. They are directed by physicians, usually pathologists or hematologists. The American Association of Blood Banks operates a clearinghouse for the exchange of blood and blood credits among hospitals.

American Blood Commission (ABC). This commission, established in 1975, is a coalition of some forty organizations representing blood banks; professionals; and consumers, including labor unions, insurers, and citizens' groups. Primary sponsors are the American Association of Blood Banks, the American National Red Cross, and the Council of Community Blood Centers. This commission was formed in response to the announcement by the Department of Health, Education and Welfare of a "national blood policy" with the goal of improving the distribution, availability, and safety of blood and its products, and with emphasis on volunteer donors.[6]

Regulation

The FDA's *Bureau of Biologics* licenses interstate blood banks. Additionally, after determining blood to be a drug in 1973, the bureau has been inspecting intrastate banks and setting standards for "good manufacturing practices."

THE MEDICAL EQUIPMENT AND SUPPLY INDUSTRY

The manufacture and distribution of supplies, medical instruments, and equipment for places such as hospitals, physicians and dentists' offices, and laboratories is an important aspect of the health care industry. These items range from laboratory glassware, needles, syringes, and dressings to complex, expensive "high technology" x-ray and electronic equipment. Their diversity is well illustrated in Table 9–3. (Additionally there is a whole range of items, from paper clips to computers, that are supplied by the general business community.) Many of the current controversial cost and ethical issues in medical care are related to equipment such as CT scanners, respirators, and renal dialysis units—technology that has become widely available.

These manufacturers and suppliers are independent for-profit companies and corporations. They vary greatly in size but there has been a trend toward consolidation, increase in size (often by merger and acquistion), and corporate diversification. Examples of large diversified companies are the American Hospital Supply Corporation and Johnson and Johnson. An example of a company specializ-

6. An important issue in the use of blood has been controlling a virus-caused hepatitis that has been shown to be more common in the blood of paid donors.

Table 9-3.   Product/Service Classifications.

Ambulances
Analytical Balances
Analytical Instrument Data Systems
Analytical Instruments
Anesthesia Equipment and Accessories
Animal Equipment and Supplies
Animal Products
Anti-embolism Devices
Appliances and Utility Equipment
Arterial Grafts
Artificial Voice Devices
Auditory Testing Equipment
Automated Cell Sorters
Automated Chemistry Analyzers
Automated Liquid Chromatography Analyzers
Automated Microbiology Analyzers
Automated RIA Systems
Automatic Slide Stainers
Beds, Specialty
Biochemicals
Biologicals
Blood and Blood Products
Blood Collection Supplies
Blood Flowmeters
Blood Gas Analyzers & Blood pH Systems
Blood Pressure Measuring Equipment
Blood Processing Equipment
Calibration and Test Equipment
Cardiac Assist Equipment
Cardiac Pacemakers
Cardiopulmonary Diagnostic Equipment
Cardiovascular Accessories
Centrifuges
Chemicals
Chromatography and Electrophoresis
  Equipment
Clinical Laboratory Products
Clinical Laboratory Testing Services
Coagulation Testing Equipment
Consulting and Planning Services
Consumable Products
Contraceptive Devices
Cryosurgical Equipment
CT Scanners
Culture Media
Data Processing Services
Defibrillators
Dental Equipment
Dental Laboratory Services
Dental Products
Dental Prosthetics
Dental Supplies
Dental X-Ray Apparatus
Diagnostic Reagents and Test Kits

Dietary, Nutritional and Vitamin Supplements
Dilutors and Dispensers
Dressings and Bandages
Electrocardiographs
Electrodes and Gels
Electroencephalographs
Electrolyte Analysis Equipment
Electromyographs
Electron Microscopes
Electronic Blood Cell Counters
Electronic Sight Aids
Electronic Thermometers
Electrosurgical Instruments
Emergency Medical Products
Employment Services
Environmentally Controlled Enclosures
Eyeglasses and Contact Lenses
Fermenters, Freeze-Dryers/Processing
  Equipment
Fiberoptic Examining Scopes
Freezers and Refrigeration Equipment
Furniture and Casework
Gas Chromatographs (Biomedical)
General Disposables
Hearing Aids
Heart Valves
Heart/Lung Machines
Holter Monitoring Services
Hospital Management Services
Hospital Supplies Distribution
Housekeeping and Laundry Services
Hyperbaric Chambers
Image Recording Systems
Implantables
Infusion Devices
Injectors
Instrument Refurbishing and Reconditioning
Instrument Repair and Maintenance
Kits and Trays
Laboratory Animals
Laboratory Data Processing Equipment
Laboratory Equipment/Supplies
Laboratory Incubators
Laboratory Ware
Laminar Flow Stations
Leasing and Rental Services
Mass Spectrometers
Material Handling Systems
Medical Building, Finance and Construction
Medical Clinic Management Services
Medical Communications Systems
Medical Data Processing Equipment
Medical Diagnostic Communications Systems
Medical Educational Services

Table 9-3. continued

Medical Educational Supplies	Pulmonary Function Testing Equipment
Medical Electronic Diagnostic Equipment	Pumps
Medical Gases and Equipment	Radiation Therapy Equipment
Medical Linens and Apparel	Radioimmunoassay Equipment
Medical Research and Development	Radioimmunoassay Test Kits
Medical Services	Radioimmunoassay Testing Services
Medical Transportation	Radioisotopes
Medical/Surgical Gloves	Radiological and Nuclear Equipment
Medical/Surgical Supplies	Radiological Monitoring Services
Microbiological and Serological Testing Equipment	Radiological Testing Services
Microporous Membrane Filters	Radiology/Nuclear Laboratory Data Systems
Microscopy Accessories	Radiopaque Contrast Media
Microtomes and Cryogenic Microtomes	Radiopharmaceuticals
Neonatal Incubators	Recorder Paper, Charts and Records
Nephrology Treatment Services	Renal Dialysis Equipment
Neurostimulators	Renal Dialysis Supplies
Nuclear Diagnostic Equipment	Respiratory Gas Analyzers
Nuclear Instruments	Respiratory Therapy Equipment
Nuclear Medical Testing Services	Respiratory Therapy Services
Nuclear Supplies and Accessories	Semen Storage
Nursing Home Management Services	Spectrophotometers, Colorimeters, Flourometers and Nephelometers
Operating Tables	Sterile Packaging Material
Ophthalmic Diagnostic Equipment	Sterilization Services
Optical Microscopes	Sterilizing Equipment
Optometric Services	Suction Machines
Orthopedic Devices and Appliances	Supply Carts and Cabinets
Other Medical Equipment	Surgical and Obstetric Drapes
Other Medical Services	Surgical Instruments
Pacemaker Batteries	Sutures and Fasteners
Parenteral and Irrigating Solutions	Syringes and Needles
Pathology Tissue Processors	Thermographic Diagnostic Equipment
Patient Monitoring Equipment	Thermometers
Patient Transport Systems	Transtelephonic EKG Analysis
Patient Weighing Equipment	Tubing, Tubes and Catheters
Patient Wheel Chairs	Ultrasonic Diagnostic Equipment
Pharmaceutical Services	Ultrasonic Transducers and Accessories
Pharmaceuticals, Drugs and Medicines	Water Treatment Equipment
Physical Therapy and Rehabilitation Equipment	X-Ray Apparatus
Physicians' Aids	X-Ray Film
Physicians' Office Testing Equipment	X-Ray Film Loading, Processing and Handling Systems
Physiological Testing Equipment and Recorders	X-Ray Supplies and Accessories
Physiological Therapeutic Equipment	X-Ray Tables
Prosthetic Devices	

Reproduced with permission from *The Medical and Healthcare Marketplace Guide*, Adeline B. Hale and Arthur B. Hale (Miami: International Bio-Medical Information Service, Inc., 1978).

ing in complex electronic patient monitoring machines is Hewlett Packard.

Under the provisions of the Medical Devices Act of 1976, various medical equipment is regulated by the FDA (through the Bureau of Medical Devices). Covered by this legislation are most laboratory equipment, implants, prostheses, artificial organs, and other products. For certain devices, as with new drugs, the manufacturer must demonstrate safety and efficiency prior to marketing.

SELECTED READINGS

"Upton Sinclair and the Pure Food and Drug Act of 1906," Arlene F. Kantor, *American Journal of Public Health* 66, no. 12 (December): 1976.

Health in a Bottle. L. Earle Arnow (Philadelphia: J. B. Lippincott Co., 1970).

Prescription Durg Industry Fact Book, Pharmaceutical Manufacturers Association. (Every 3-4 years). Pharmaceuticals, medical devices and diagnostic products.

Pills, Profits and Politics, Milton Silverman and Philip R. Lee (Berkeley: University of California Press, 1974). This is the best source. The authors work hard to present both sides of the major issues, which is a rarity in the literature on the drug industry.

"The Drug Regulation Process and the Challenge of Regulatory Reform," Norman Dorsen and Jeffry M. Miller, *Annals of Internal Medicine* 91, no. 6 (December): 908-913.

The Gift Relationship: From Human Blood to Social Policy, Richard M. Titmuss (New York: Vintage Books, 1971).

Economic Organization in Medical Equipment and Supply, R.D. Peterson and C.R. MacPhee (Lexington, Massachusetts: Lexington Books, 1973).

Policy Implications of the Computed Tomography (CT) Scanner, Office of Technology Assessment, United States Congress (Washington, D.C.: U.S. Government Printing Office, 1978).

10 REVIEW AND CONTROL OF QUALITY AND COSTS

REVIEW AND CONTROL OF QUALITY

Activities related to the maintenance of quality in health care may be considered under three general categories:

- *Licensure* of manpower and facilities by government agencies.
- Voluntary *accreditation* of institutions and programs and *certification* of competence of personnel by professional organizations.
- Detailed review of the many dimensions of health care by a variety of methods under the rubrics of *medical audit* and *quality assurance.*

Licensure

The states exercise extensive licensing powers for health manpower and institutions, including continuing regulation of licensees. By appropriate legislation, they may authorize persons who meet stated educational and, usually, examination criteria to engage in certain health occupations and professions. In addition to setting forth the general criteria, the legislation usually establishes boards of licensure or registration to implement the provisions, make rules and regulations, and set procedures. Such boards are made up in large part of members of the profession being licensed.

257

As of 1977, thirty-five health occupations were licensed in one or more states (see page 64). The stimulus for licensure has often come from professional groups and is sometimes viewed as one manifestation of the process of "professionalization" of health occupations. Another stimulus is exemplified by the rapid requirement by all states of licensure of nursing home administrators. Such licensure was federally mandated as of 1970[1] for state participation in Medicaid.

In addition to such regulation of manpower, the states also license hospitals and other health care institutions. In most cases this authority is vested by the legislature in the state health department. In some instances it is delegated to local city or county authorities. Hospitals are licensed in all states (except general hospitals in Ohio). Nursing homes and pharmacies are licensed in all states.

Accreditation

Accreditation is the process by which an institution or an educational program is determined to meet certain generally accepted standards set forth by an appropriate professional association. It is voluntary, and an institution or program must apply to the accrediting agency for the necessary appraisal. Accrediting bodies are generally composed of representatives of professional organizations concerned with the institutions or programs in question and their titles (council, committee, commission, etc.) generally reflect their collaborative purpose. In addition to organizations represented on the governing bodies, others may participate in cooperative and advisory capacities.

The most important example of an institutional accrediting body is the Joint Commission on Accreditation of Hospitals (JCAH). The JCAH had its origin in a resolution of the 1912 Third Clinical Congress of Surgeons in North America, which recommended that "some system of standardization of hospital equipment and hospital wards should be developed." The Congress was influenced by the 1910 publication of the "Flexner report" on medical school deficiencies (see page 261) and proposals were made for an analogous survey of hospitals.[2] The first hospital survey was carried out in 1918 by the

---

1. Under the 1967 Social Security amendments.

2. Discussions of the historical origin of the JCAH may be found in *Evolution of the Medical Audit*, Paul Lembeke (see Selected Readings, p. 272) and in "American Surgery's Noblest Experiment," Carl F. Schlicke, *Archives of Surgery* 106 (1973): 379–385.

newly established American College of Surgeons. This effort evolved into the JCAH, which was formed in 1951 by the American College of Surgeons, American College of Physicians, American Hospital Association, American Medical Association, and Canadian Medical Association. The Canadians withdrew in 1959 to found their own accrediting body. The American Dental Association became a member in 1979.

The JCAH develops standards and provides advice to hospitals about meeting them. A hospital seeking accreditation must be accepted for registration by the American Hospital Association (AHA), request a survey by a JCAH survey team, and pay a fee. The hospital is accredited for up to three years, or not accredited. Approximately 5,000 hospitals are accredited by the JCAH, including virtually all those with over 100 beds.

In addition to the accreditation of short-term acute care hospitals that forms the bulk of its work, the JCAH also accredits long-term care facilities, psychiatric facilities, and ambulatory care programs. Standards are developed with the participation of interested professional organizations and voluntary agencies.[3]

A 1979 internal reorganization of the JCAH replaced its accreditation councils with a professional and technical advisory committee for each accreditation program. In this context independent organizations were formed for the accreditation of ambulatory care programs—the *Accreditation Association for Ambulatory Health Care*—and facilities for the mentally retarded—the *Accreditation Council for Services for Mentally Retarded and Other Developmentally Disabled Persons.*

Examples of accreditation bodies for educational institutions are the *Liaison Committee on Medical Education* (a joint committee of the American Medical Association (AMA) and the Association of American Medical Colleges), which accredits medical schools; and the *Council on Education for Public Health* (American Public Health

---

3. For example, in 1981 the committee concerned with standards for psychiatric facilities included representation from the American Association of Psychiatric Services for Children, National Association of State Alcohol and Drug Abuse Directors, American Hospital Association, American Occupational Therapy Association, American Nurses' Association, National Association of State Mental Health Program Directors, National Association of Private Psychiatric Hospitals, American Psychiatric Association, National Association of Social Workers, Association of Mental Health Administrators, American Academy of Child Psychiatry, National Coalition for Alcoholism Program Accreditation, National Council of Community Mental Health Centers, and the American Psychological Association.

Association and Association of Schools of Public Health), which accredits schools of public health.

Specific educational programs may also be accredited. For example, the National League for Nursing separately accredits nursing education programs at the diploma school, associate degree, baccalaureate, and masters degree levels, and the Association of University Programs in Health Administration[4] participates in the accreditation of programs in health administration.

There is a large number of other accrediting programs sponsored by various professional associations. The percentages of entities seeking accreditation varies considerably. With some, the process is quasi-voluntary, in that accreditation has important financial implications in addition to organizational prestige. For example, in the case of hospitals, accreditation is required for reimbursement by many insurance plans, including Blue Cross; and accredited hospitals are deemed to have fulfilled most Medicare participation requirements. Educational programs also need accreditation for eligibility for federal grants and student financial assistance programs. (For the purpose of such federal funding the Department of Education lists officially recognized accrediting bodies.)

Certification

Certification (or *registration*), is the voluntary process by which individual health personnel are affirmed to have attained a certain level of qualification, according to standards and criteria such as education, experience, and examination, as set forth by their professional associations. These may be basic criteria for recognition of individuals as qualified to engage in the occupation, or may be criteria for recognition of advanced qualifications or specialization. An example of the former is the certification of inhalation therapy technicians by the American Association for Inhalation Therapy; examples of the latter are the many medical specialists certified by specialty boards such as those affiliated with the American Academy of Internal Medicine, the American Academy of Pediatrics, and the American College of Surgeons (see also Chapter 4). Not all otherwise qualified health personnel seek certification; the numbers who do

---

4. Formerly the Association of University Programs in Hospital Administration.

vary considerably and are apt to be higher in categories where such certification enhances employment and practice opportunities and income levels. Many professional groups offer recertification examinations. In some instances, such periodic recertification is required (for example, the American Board of Family Practice).

The term "registration" may refer, depending on the context, to both licensure and certification. Boards of licensure and certification boards are both often termed boards of registration or registries; also, the terms "license" and "certificate of registration" are often used interchangeably.

Continuing Education. Continuing education is actively encouraged by many professional societies; some have developed formal self-study programs, often geared to certification and (largely voluntary) recertification. Increasingly, states are mandating participation in continuing education for maintenance of licensure. For physicians, the continuing medical education (CME) system often used is modeled after that developed by the American Medical Association, which sets forth five categories of educational activities. (Category I, the most emphasized, includes formal conferences and courses sponsored by organizations accredited for CME by the *Accreditation Council for Continuing Medical Education*.[5] Another widely used system is the *continuing education unit* (CEU) system in which one unit is given for each ten hours of attendance at a recognized educational program.

Medical Audit (Quality Assessment)

In addition to these widely prevalent official and quasi-official mechanisms described above, the problem of evaluation and control of the quality of medical care has been addressed in many other ways since the publication in 1910 of the most widely known single quality study, the Carnegie Foundation's Flexner Report[6] on medical education. This nationwide survey of medical schools documented many serious deficiencies of the schools (including the many proprietary

---

5. Sponsored by the Association of American Medical Colleges, American Board of Medical Specialties, Council of Medical Specialty Societies, American Hospital Association, Federation of State Medical Boards, and Association for Hospital Medical Education.

6. See *Medical Education in the United States and Canada* (Selected Readings, p. 272).

institutions that existed at the time) and contributed significantly to subsequent reforms.

Most of these quality assessment efforts have been variations on the technique of *medical audit*, which may be broadly defined as the appraisal of quality by medical record review. This commonly has taken the form of analyses of individual cases, with judgments based on defined criteria (*explicit criteria*) for diagnosis and management, on expert opinion (*implicit criteria*), or on a combination of these.[7] Medical audits may be *internal* (developed and carried out by an organization's own staff) or *external* (carried out by outside reviewers).

The terms "quality assessment," "quality appraisal," and "medical audit" are often used interchangeably. Some consider "quality assessment" a broader term, with "medical audit" connoting a narrower focus on individual review. Others prefer the older term "medical audit" for the general process of evaluation of quality. The term "quality assurance" implies a program designed not only to assess quality but to alter professional and organizational behavior so as to remedy deficiencies and improve performance.

Three major dimensions of quality review are now widely accepted: *structure* (organizational setting, physical resources, and manpower attributes); *process* (activities and decisions of health professionals in patient care); and *outcome* (end results).[8] Additional dimensions commonly accepted are *accessibility of care* and *patient satisfaction*. Outcome measurements have attracted particular recent research interest.

Professional Activity Study (PAS). The Professional Activity Study was begun in 1953 by the Southwestern Michigan Hospital Council to develop methods to compare medical practices among hospitals. It is now conducted by the Commission on Professional and Hospi-

---

7. This case analysis technique was first exemplified by the surgical "end results" studies of Ernest A. Codman in Boston from 1912 to 1916 and has again been widely used since interest in assessing quality redeveloped around 1950. (Codman's work is described in his *Studies in Hospital Efficiency*, privately published in Boston c. 1917. His studies considerably influenced the deliberations that led to the 1918 hospital survey of the New American College of Surgeons.)

8. They were conceptually described and discussed by Donabedian in 1966 in *Evaluating the Quality of Medical Care* (see Selected Readings).

tal Activities (CPHA).[9] This program, under its first director Virgil Slee, pioneered the application of data processing techniques (first mechanical, then electronic) to the collection and analyses of medical record information on a large scale. Under this program, medical record personnel of participating hospitals abstract standard data from patient records at the time of hospital discharge. The data so obtained is then processed and reported to the hospital in the form of statistical summaries and case-by-case tabulations. Over 1,500 hospitals nationwide now participate in PAS. The Medical Audit Program (MAP) is a related program whereby data are tabulated by clinical service in such a way as to facilitate review of patterns of professional practice. Many hospitals use the PAS health data system in connection with their utilization review activities (see below).

REVIEW AND CONTROL OF COSTS

The control of health care costs has become a dominant concern. Many approaches have been used including those involving review of individual utilization of services (claims review and utilization review), control of capital expenditures such as construction of facilities and acquisition of expensive equipment, the use of budgetary and reimbursement controls, the promotion of system components deemed cost-effective, and the promotion of competition in general.

Utilization Control and Utilization Review (UR)

Control of the use of medical services has generally been considered an important dimension of cost control. Most of the formal activity in this area has been by some form of *utilization review*, which essentially involves the assessment of the necessity for medical services. This has come to be an important aspect of attempts to control Medicare and Medicaid expenditures. It has been largely directed to institutional services, particularly hospital admissions, and involves the review of patient hospitalizations to determine the necessity of the admissions and to monitor lengths of stay and use of services.

---

9. Under the sponsorship of the American College of Physicians, the American College of Surgeons, the American Hospital Association, and the Southwestern Michigan Hospital Council.

Hospital Utilization Committees. It had long been a practice, especially during and after World War II, for the medical staffs of some hospitals with shortages of available beds and manpower to establish committees to monitor admissions, including the setting of priorities. About 1960, however, the number of such committees began to increase, now largely under the pressures of health insurers, due to the rising costs of hospital care.

The most widely noted early example of such pressures was the 1958 order of the Pennsylvania insurance commissioner to three Pennsylvania Blue Cross plans (which had requested rate increases) that steps must be taken to control costs. This led to the establishment of utilization committees in many Pennsylvania hospitals. (The term "utilization review" is said to have first been used by these committees.) Their experience contributed to the establishment of similar committees in other hospitals.

The Hospital Utilization Project of Pennsylvania (HUP), sponsored by the Allegheny County Medical Society and the Hospital Council of Western Pennsylvania, was established in 1963 as a pilot project to provide centralized assistance to the Pennsylvania review committees by providing computerized information on hospital discharges. It provided important early experience in the use of such regional computerized data for utilization review. About 700 hospitals in 30 states now use the expanded HUP health data system.

The Medicare legislation (Social Security Amendments of 1965) required that participating hospitals and extended care facilities have *utilization review plans.* This stipulation led to the formation of utilization review committees in all these institutions as well as to considerable interest in the general problems of such review. The 1972 Social Security Amendments provided for the establishment of *professional standards review organizations,* to review services provided under the Medicare and Medicaid programs (see page 270). For the majority of hospitals, such review has been delegated to hospital utilization review committees under PSRO supervision.[10]

Initially, the hospital committees were largely geared to educating physicians about appropriate hospital use and identifying administrative factors contributing to prolongation of hospital stays. Increasingly, however, financial sanctions have been imposed on patients

---

10. Some hospitals have consolidated their utilization review and quality assurance programs together with other preventive legal measures under a *risk management* program.

and hospitals by denial of payments for all or part of hospital stays deemed unnecessary.[11]

General Terms. The process of utilization review and control now encompasses a variety of procedures, including:

Certification: A written statement by an admitting physician affirming the necessity of a hospital admission, or a statement of approval of admission by authorized reviewers (preadmission certification).[12]

Concurrent review: The monitoring (by the UR Committee) during the course of a hospital stay, usually with emphasis on extended stays, such as over thirty days.

Retrospective review: A review after the discharge of the patient or elapse of the covered benefit period.

Prior review: A review at or near the time of admission, or (by the insurer) in advance of admission, such as in the case of elective surgery or a nursing home admission. These are then generally considered *certified admissions*, with payment guaranteed for at least a set period of time. This has been a controversial procedure and is not widely used for general hospital admissions. It has, however, mitigated some of the problems associated with "retroactive denial" of reimbursements for nursing home care.

Second opinion: A consultation by a second surgical consultant regarding the need for proposed elective surgery. It is usually a voluntary program, and the fees for such consultations are paid by the insurance company or by Medicaid.

---

11. In the case of utilization review in nursing homes, emphasis is less on necessity of admission than on whether the status of the patient meets criteria for coverage set by Medicare or the insurance company, or whether the patient is in the proper level of care (see pages 36 and 39).

12. Admission certification was an early form of utilization control. For example, in 1955, New Jersey Blue Cross introduced a system whereby admissions were initially approved for twenty-eight days (later fourteen days) and reapproved at twenty-one-day (later fourteen-day),intervals. A program of approval by individual diagnosis was begun in 1965.

Control of Capital Expenditures

Among the more controversial mechanisms of cost control are those directed toward control of capital expenditures.

Health Planning Agencies. There has been in every state except Rhode Island one or more area-wide *health systems agencies* (HSAs), generally nonprofit corporations; a state *health planning and coordinating agency*; and a statewide *health coordinating council*. The system was established under the federal National Health Planning and Development Act of 1974 and superseded the previous comprehensive health planning "314a" and "314b" agencies established under 1966 health planning legislation. (These had previously supplanted the health and hospital planning councils, established in the context of the Hill–Burton hospital construction grants program, and other voluntary planning groups.[13]) The purpose of these agencies is to develop local and state plans, including the collection of relevant data, for the appropriate development of health resources. They approve applications for federal funds under many grant-in-aid programs and are generally involved in the states' certificate of need programs. Each health systems agency is responsible for one of the 203 *health service areas* that have not been designated nationwide, one or more in each state, according to population. There has been disagreement as to the effectiveness of the HSAs and their future is problematical. For example, under the 1981 federal budget legislation states may request that health planning activities under the federal program be carried out at the state level only, with elimination of the HSAs. The state of Ohio was the first to take such action. The *American Health Planning Association* is the national organization for health planners.

"Certificate of Need" Statutes. "Certificate of need" (CON) or "determination of need" (DON) statutes are state-enacted legislation whose primary purpose is the control of capital expenditures by health facilities. They have been directed particularly at hospital and nursing home construction but, variably according to state, cover

13. Many of these older groups evolved into the present planning agencies, often by a complex political process.

other aspects of the health system, including ambulatory care facilities and the acquisition of expensive equipment.[14] In general, under these statutes, construction, renovations, and (variably) new services and equipment costing more than $150,000 must be approved by a designated state agency (usually the state health department or board), often with the concurrence of the local health systems agency.[15] Evidence that the new or expanded facility or service is needed by the community must be presented.

The first such legislation was enacted by New York state in 1964, and was followed by Maryland and Rhode Island in 1968. As of 1981, virtually all states had such statutes, a trend accelerated by the 1974 federal health planning legislation that mandated the enactment of such state statutes as a condition of receiving certain federal grant funds.

Section 1122 Reviews. Another example of an attempt at capital expenditure control was Section 1122 of the 1972 Social Security Amendments, which permitted the states to designate state agencies to review proposed capital expenditures by health organizations. The statutory penalty for construction deemed unneeded was a reduction in allowed depreciation under the Medicare reimbursement formula. This program is not generally considered to have been very effective.

Control of Reimbursement Rates and Budgets

This type of cost control operates through the regulation of funds disbursed to institutional providers of care.

Prospective Reimbursement. *Prospective reimbursement* is a general term for mechanisms of payment for institutional health care services at a rate determined in advance, as opposed to the traditional method of reimbursement after the fact (*retrospective reimbursement, cost reimbursement*) for costs incurred. Negotiated rates of payment are established in advance, yearly, and paid regardless of

14. The most celebrated example of such "high technology" equipment, is the *computed axial tomography scanner* (CAT, CT scanner) an important, very expensive advance in diagnostic radiology.

15. The relationship between the health planning agencies and the certificate of need process varies from state to state.

costs actually incurred. A number of states have established public rate-setting bodies (rate-setting commissions, cost control commissions). Programs have also been established by many Blue Cross plans.[16]

There have also been some experimental *incentive reimbursement* programs whereby savings developed by various methods are shared by the insurer and the organization. (Some use the term "incentive reimbursement" instead of "prospective reimbursement," considering that prospective reimbursement provides inherent incentives for cost control.)

Another budgetary control device is the *revenue cap* — a prominent feature of proposed federal cost containment legislation whereby hospital charges would be limited to a fixed annual percentage increase. An experimental program in Rhode Island has provided for a limit on total allowable expense increases statewide (MAXICAP) with hospital budgets individually negotiated within this limit.

Diagnosis-Related Groups. A relatively new system of reimbursement involves *diagnosis-related groups* (DRGs), whereby payment is related to the type of illness being paid for, an acknowledgment of the different "case mix" found in different hospitals. DRG systems classify 383 types of cases seen in acute care hospitals. Subgroups take into account factors such as age and complications. A number of cost control commissions have incorporated this system into their programs.

Promotion of Competition

The encouragement of increased competition in the marketplace is advocated by some economists and regulators as a means of cost containment.

One example is the encouragement of the presumed cost-effective health maintenance organizations (HMOs), whose presence is thought to exert salutory influences on other components of the health system. (See Chapter 5.)

---

16. Payment at a preset rate has long been a feature of payment for noninstitutional services, particularly by public agencies. Set Medicaid payments for visits to ambulatory facilities, and fee schedules for physician services under Workman's Compensation and Blue Shield plans are examples.

The Federal Trade Commission (FTC) has been taking a number of steps to control alleged anticompetitive practices in medical and related practices. Several professional societies have signed consent decrees under which they have abandoned their relative value scales, deemed to be price fixing.[17] The FTC has also directed the AMA to refrain from the prohibition (in its code of ethics) of advertising by physicians, has prohibited restrictions on advertising eyeglass prices, has argued against physician dominance of Blue Shield boards, and has warned physicians against impeding the development of HMOs.

COMBINED APPROACHES TO UTILIZATION AND QUALITY REVIEW

There has been a general trend toward the integration of techniques for the systematic review of quality and utilization of services. In these approaches considerations of cost control dominate. (Some have argued, however, that the appropriate use of resources is in itself an attribute of good quality.) Among many examples of the trend is the use of PAS data by utilization review groups.

Foundations for Medical Care (Medical Care Foundations) [18]

Foundations for medical care are independent nonprofit physician-sponsored corporations that provide one or more services related to third-party payments to participating physicians. Declared common goals are the peer review of costs and quality of care in a fee-for-service context.

All foundations perform some type of review and monitoring of services. Such activities range from review of claims referred by third-party payers (Blue Cross–Blue Shield, and commercial insurance carriers) to the development of norms for medical procedures, hospitalizations, and length of stay for selected diagnoses. Some foundations sponsor prepaid health insurance plans (health main-

---

17. The American Society of Anesthesiologists has successfully contested a similar order by the Department of Justice's antitrust division, while acceding to a FTC order to cease prohibiting the salaried (versus fee-for-services) practice by hospital-based anesthesiologists.

18. Despite the similar terminology, these should not be confused with philanthropic formulations (described on p. 241).

tenance organizations) through individual practice associations (IPAs), for which they provide complete claims processing, and review and monitoring. (See Chapter 5.)

Most of the development of such foundations has taken place since 1965, and much of this since 1970, although the original organization, the San Joaquin Foundation for Medical Care, was established in 1954. (This was the prototype for the foundations that sponsor complete prepaid health insurance plans.) The relationship between foundations for medical care and state and county medical societies varies from formal medical society sponsorship to complete independence.

A number of preexisting foundations became designated as professional standards review organizations for their areas. (Other foundations were established for the specific purpose of being so designated. Many of these are developing broader activities and are thus becoming more like the older foundations.)

The *American Association of Foundations for Medical Care* gathers and distributes information about these organizations.

Peer Review. This term is often used for the general process of medical review of utilization and quality, when this is carried out directly or under the supervision of physicians; it often carries the implication that these will be practicing physicians.

Professional Standards Review Organizations (PSROs)

The establishment of *professional standards review organizations* was mandated by the Social Security Amendments of 1972 (Medicare–Medicaid amendments). They are associations of physicians that review professional and institutional services provided under the Medicare and Medicaid programs. The stated purpose is the monitoring and control of both cost and quality, although they have been evaluated by Congress in terms of their effectiveness in cost control.

In mid–1981 there were 182 federally funded PSROs. Many were developed through state or local medical society auspices, sometimes through foundations for medical care; others were established independently. Twenty-eight PSROs were statewide. The other states had two to five PSRO areas.

In the majority of instances, PSRO review functions for hospitals have been delegated to hospital utilization review committees that have been deemed capable and willing to carry out effective review. (Medical audit committees, usually separate, are also mandated.) Occasionally these functions have been "de-delegated" and resumed by the PSRO.

In addition to their Medicare and Medicaid review activities an increasing number of PSROs are performing review functions for health insurance companies and industrial corporations concerned about controlling costs of their employee health insurance plans. Such nongovernmental review activities, as noted above, have been carried out for some time by the older foundations for medical care.

The number of federally funded PSROs has been decreasing, a decline that is being accelerated by more stringent funding criteria in the setting of the Reagan administration's federal budget reductions. (Recommendations by the administration for their total elimination were not accepted by Congress.)

The *American Association of Professional Standards Review Organizations* addresses the interests of these organizations.

Experimental Medical Review Organizations (EMCROs). This term was applied to ten foundations for medical care and other medical society-sponsored review organizations that participated, beginning in 1971, in a program sponsored and funded by the National Center for Health Services Research and Development, to develop models for the systematic review of physician services. The EMCRO program was developed in anticipation of the PSRO provisions of the 1972 Social Security Amendments. These experimental, research-oriented projects tended to be relatively comprehensive, often addressing nursing home, office care, and use of drugs as well as hospital care. Most of these organizations became the PSROs for their areas.

Cost control is one of the most rapidly changing aspects of the health care system. There is much disagreement over whether extensive regulatory control, directly or indirectly by government, or the promotion of competition "in the marketplace" is the more effective policy. Under the Reagan administration there has been much advocacy of strategies to increase competition.

SELECTED READINGS

Medical Education in the United States and Canada, a report to the Carnegie Foundation for the Advancement of Teaching, Abraham Flexner (New York: The Carnegie Foundation, 1910).

"Evolution of the Medical Audit," Paul A. Lembcke, *Journal of the American Medical Association* 199 (1967): 111.

"Evaluating the Quality of Medical Care," Avedis Donabedian, *Milbank Memorial Fund Quarterly* XLIV (1966): 166.

Explorations in Quality Assessment and Monitoring, Volumes I and II, Avedis Donabedian [Ann Arbor: Health Administration Press, 1980 (Vol. I) and 1982 (Vol. II)].

Medical Technology: The Culprit Behind Health Care Costs, Stuart A. Altman and Robert Blensley, eds. Proceedings of the 1977 Sun Valley Forum on National Health (Department of Health, Education and Welfare, Public Health Service, 1979).

Regulating Health Care: The Struggle for Control. Proceedings of the Academy of Political Science, Arthur Levin, ed. (New York: The Academy of Political Science, 1980).

"The Health Planners and Computerized Tomography: High Technology, Cost Control, and Judicial Review," William J. Curran, *New England Journal of Medicine* 303, (1980): 62667.

"Certificate of Need: Theory and Experience" in *Deregulating the Health Care Industry*, Clark Havighurst (Cambridge, Massachusetts: Ballinger Publishing Company).

"Foundations for Medical Care," Richard H. Egdahl, *New England Journal of Medicine* 288 (1973): 491.

"The PSRO in Perspective," Helen L. Smits, *New England Journal of Medicine* 305 (1981): 253.

11 HEALTH LAW AND MEDICAL ETHICS

The fields of health law and medical ethics are large, very complex, and expanding. The purpose of this chapter is simply to briefly review the more important concepts, issues, and terminology.

Law (there are many definitions) can be viewed as the rules set forth for the governing and social control of human societies, rules that have been or are subject to adjudication in the courts. It is the special domain of lawyers, jurists, legislators, and administrators.

Ethics has to do with the concept of right and wrong, of morality. It has traditionally been the domain of philosophers and theologians and has been called "moral philosophy."

The two areas are of course interrelated and this has become particularly the case in the health system.

Health law is a broad term covering law as it relates to the entire health field. The terms *legal medicine, forensic medicine,* and the frequently used adjective *medico-legal* are often used in the context of medicine and medical practice. The term health law has also sometimes been used to refer more specifically to public health law.

Medical ethics (*biomedical ethics, bioethics*) has come to particular prominence with the increasing importance of biomedical research and technology.

THE LEGAL STRUCTURE

The legal structure of the United States has several components.

Constitutional Law

The U.S. Constitution, adopted by the states in 1789, is the supreme law of the land and all other law, including the state constitutions, must be consistent with it. Under the Constitution certain powers were given by the states to the federal government with all other powers reserved to the states. The words "health" and "medicine" do not appear in the Constitution. Nevertheless, the federal government has developed many important activities related to health through the exercise of constitutional powers to regulate interstate and foreign commerce and to promote the general welfare. (See Chapter 6.) The states have separate constitutions with which their laws must be consistent. Court suits based upon "due process" are based on constitutional law.[1]

Statutory Law

Laws passed by legislative bodies are termed *statutes* (or in the case of local law, *ordinances*). These are compiled in statutory *codes*. The states pass a wide variety of laws under the inherent "police power" of the sovereign state to take actions protecting the general health, safety, and welfare of the public. (See Chapter 7.)

Administrative Law

Administrative law encompasses the rules and regulations by which statutes are carried out or implemented by administrative agencies or through which specific regulatory agencies carry out their work. (See also page 000.)

---

1. The fifth and fourteenth amendments to the Constitution provide that individuals may not be deprived of life, liberty, or property without due process of law.

Common Law (Case Law)

Common law is law that has been developed from court cases based on precedent and custom. It is derived from English common law. Most *civil actions*, actions by one person or group against another, are carried out under common law. Among the types of civil suits that can be brought are those related to *contracts* (for example, breach of contract) and those involving wrongful acts or *torts* that involve injury through infringement on personal or property rights. The most frequent and well-known cause for the latter type of civil action in the health field is *professional negligence* or "malpractice" (See below.)

THE LAW AND HEALTH INSTITUTIONS

Health institutions, such as hospitals, exist by authority of the states under general statutes regarding *corporations* or by specific statutes or *charters*.[2]

Corporations.   The law of each state determines the existence of corporations in that state, and defines requirements for corporate status. For-profit and not-for-profit corporations are distinguished by the Federal Internal Revenue Code, which defines the tax status of corporations. A nonprofit organization can engage to some extent in for-profit activities outside its corporate purpose and can be taxed on those profits. Nonprofit corporations are managed by trustees who do not usually receive pay for their work. Trustees have a fiduciary responsibility to their organization; that is, they must act in the interests of that organization.

Additionally, hospitals are licensed by the states to provide health services and are the subject of a large and increasing number of governmental regulatory activities, both state and federal. These include regulations related to Medicare and Medicaid, cost control, rate setting, and many others.

As corporate entities, health institutions are subject to civil actions, including suits for *negligence*. In the past, public and nonprofit

2. Exceptions are federal institutions; these are not regulated by the states.

organizations had *government immunity* and *charitable immunity* from law suits, but this has been disappearing, especially for non-profit organizations. Institutions, including hospitals have long been held responsible for actions of their employees,[3] but court decisions in recent years have widened the scope of hospital responsibility for the quality of care rendered by its nonemployee physician staff, such responsibility to be carried out through appropriate procedures and mechanisms, including the organized medical staff and staff bylaws.[4]

Hospitals and other health organizations, in the context of rising insurance claims and premiums have been developing organized programs of *risk management* aimed at preventing incidents that may lead to litigation. These programs include attention to recordkeeping, incident reporting, patient grievances, and quality assurance procedures.

The relationship between health institutions and their professional staffs are spelled out in corporation and staff bylaws. These relationships as they involve staff appointments and admitting privileges have been the subject of "due process" actions that have resulted in a considerable body of law on this subject.

THE LAW AND MEDICAL PRACTICE (PROFESSIONAL PRACTICE)

Practice by physicians, as well as many other professionals, is sanctioned by society through the states by *licensure laws*. In addition, certain aspects of practice are variably regulated by the states through laws concerning professional corporations, drug prescribing (for example, encouraging prescriptions of generic drugs and controlling drugs commonly abused), patient's access to their medical records, and so forth.

The physician–patient relationship is legally recognized.[5] Although a physician is not required to accept any patient for care, once such

---

3. Under the doctrine of *respondeat superior*.

4. One such case that has been often quoted and commented upon was a 1965 Illinois Supreme Court decision, *Darling* versus *Charleston Community Hospital*. It involved negligence in the treatment of a leg fracture (which led to leg amputation) by a member of the hospital's medical staff working in the emergency room under an on-call rotation.

5. The circumstances under which a physician–patient relationship is held to exist have been elucidated through many court cases.

care is undertaken the physician is expected to practice with due care and in accordance with accepted professional standards, not unilaterally terminate the relationship without appropriate notice, guard the patient's confidentiality, and carry out procedures and operations with elements of risk only with the patient's *informed consent.*

A physician may be sued on grounds similar to those in general civil actions, including *breach of contract*, if he or she can be shown to have promised results that were not forthcoming, or for *assault and battery* for procedures or operations performed without proper consent. However, the major type of legal action to which physicians and other professionals are subject is *professional negligence* or "malpractice." Physicians and other professionals may also be subject to criminal action for fraud for actions such as claiming reimbursement for services not performed (e.g., from Medicare and Medicaid).

Malpractice

Professional negligence, generally known as malpractice, is the breach of the standard of care due to the patient. It may be grounds for civil action if the negligent act (of omission or commission) caused harm or injury to the patient. Malpractice insurance (professional liability insurance) is insurance against the costs of litigation and awards. The cost of premiums, presumably reflecting increasing claims and amounts of awards, have been rapidly rising, particularly for physicians. This has varied greatly by state, premiums in California being particularly high, and by specialty, with surgical specialties the highest. The setting of premiums is complicated by the fact that it may be some years after the event before a case is finally decided by a court. Recently some groups of physicians (and hospitals) have formed their own insurance plans (called *sponsored insurance plans*). Some physicians, because of high premiums, have stopped purchasing malpractice insurance. This is called "going bare."

All of the states, responding to a perceived "malpractice insurance crisis" have in the past few years enacted various laws relating to medical malpractice litigation. These have included changes in statutes of limitation (time within which suits must be brought), ceilings on total awards, provision for pretrial screening of cases by special panels, or for binding arbitration. Many of these statutes have been and are being challenged and some have been declared unconstitutional by state courts.

"Good Samaritan Laws." Because the fear of suit has been said to deter some physicians from stopping to help accident victims or acutely ill persons, a number of states have passed laws protecting physicians from suits for negligence arising from such care.

Contingent Fee. The lawyer who successfully argues a malpractice case is usually paid a percentage of the award, called a contingent fee. The appropriateness of this method of payment has been a subject of some contention between the legal and medical profession.

Locality Rule. Traditionally, questions of professional negligence have been judged against accepted local standards (community standards) of practice. Increasingly, professionals, particularly specialists, are being held to wider, often national, standards.

"No-Fault Insurance." Some form of "no-fault" insurance has been advocated as a solution to the many problems associated with malpractice litigation. Payment to a patient or family would be made on the basis of injury or harm without the requirement of a finding of negligence.

"Defensive Medicine." It is widely believed (although little documented) that the fear of malpractice suits has led physicians to order tests and perform procedures that are not medically necessary for the purpose of defense against possible suit.

THE LAW AND MENTAL HEALTH

The law as applied to the field of mental health has become particularly prominent due to recent interest in the civil rights of the mentally ill and mentally retarded. The many issues involved are extremely complicated. What follows is a brief review of some of the more frequently encountered issues and terminology.

Mental Health and the Criminally Accused

The question of the mental competency of the criminally accused to stand trial has been addressed for many years by the courts. State laws prescribe procedures for such determinations ("sanity hearings"). The expert opinions of physicians, usually psychiatrists, are used and are an aspect of *forensic psychiatry*. The standards for mental competency include the ability of the accused to understand the nature of the proceedings against him or her and to cooperate in legal defense.

At trial, a defendant may plead not guilty by reason of insanity. The trial then involves a determination of whether the defendant was criminally responsible for the wrongful act. Generally, this is decided according to the "M'Naghten rule" regarding the understanding of right and wrong.[6] Other standards have been proposed but this rule remains the general one.

Institutional Commitment of the Mentally Ill

Civil commitment is the involuntary hospitalization of the mentally ill. In recent years the requirements and procedures for this have been made more stringent by state legislatures and by the courts in order to protect the rights of these persons. In general, mentally ill persons may be committed to mental institutions only if in the opinion of one or more physicians (commonly two) they pose a danger to themselves or others. Although some argue that reforms have gone too far and prevent the hospitalization of patients who would benefit from treatment, the issues have generally been decided in favor of the patients' civil rights.

More stringent procedures are also being required for those committed through the criminal justice system as a result of sanity hearings and insanity verdicts. The question of subsequent release of persons so committed is an often controversial one.

6. The M'Naghten rule, so named from a case decided in England in 1843, states that a defendant is not criminally responsible for an act if he was "laboring under such a defect of reason from disease of the mind as not to know the nature and quality of the act he was doing, or if he did know it, that he did not know he was doing what was wrong." Quoted in "The Physician and the Law: Determination of Mental Competency to Stand Trial," by C. B. Scrignar, *Journal of the American Medical Association*, August 7, 1967, p. 83.

The Rights of the Institutionalized Mentally Ill and Mentally Retarded

There has been considerable litigation directed to broadening the rights of those involuntarily confined in mental hospitals and those residing in institutions for the mentally retarded. The many matters addressed include the right to treatment and education of the mentally retarded, the right of the mentally ill to refuse medication and other treatment, rights related to participation in research experiments, and rights related to general living conditions. Although many questions remain unresolved there have been improvements in conditions and procedures in many state institutions and legal action has helped spread the trend toward deinstitutionalization, especially of the mentally retarded.[7]

FORENSIC PATHOLOGY

State laws provide for the investigation of sudden, suspicious, or violent death. In the past this has been the responsibility of officials called *coroners* (sometimes but not necessarily physicians), usually elected by counties or municipalities. In many jurisdictions coroners have been replaced by a system of *medical examiners*, physicians with experience in forensic medicine. Some medical examiners are trained in the specialty of *forensic pathology* (a subspecialty of pathology). There are relatively few of these specialists but their numbers are growing.

CITATION OF COURT DECISIONS

Most opinions (decisions) of the state appellate courts are generally published in the National Reporter System (West Publishing Company), which includes seven Regional Reporters and two separate reports for New York and California (Atlantic, North Eastern, North

---

7. For example, a 1975 consent decree involving New York State and public interest groups provided for residents of Willowbrook State School to be dispersed to suitable community facilities. (A consent decree is a judicially sanctioned agreement between the parties to litigation.)

Western, Pacific, South Eastern, Southern, and South Western Reporters, the California Reporter, and the New York Supplement). The states also publish their own official court opinions or in some cases designate a private publication (for example, the National Reporter). Federal court opinions are published in several official and unofficial publications including the National Reporter System's Federal Reporter and Supreme Court Reporter. Court decisions are cited by reference to these publications. For example the decision *Darling* vs. *Charleston Community Hospital* may be cited as 211 N.E.2nd 53 (1965), referring to the North Eastern Reporter, volume 211, second series, page 53. The official state publication may also be cited as 33 Ill. 2nd 326; as may be reference to the refusal of the Supreme Court to hear an appeal, *cert. denied*, 383 U.S. 946 (1966), referring to the denial of "certiorari," formal acceptance by the Court, as reported in the official U.S. Supreme Court reports.

MEDICAL ETHICS

Ethics in the medical field has in the past largely been addressed in the context of codes of professional behavior (for example, the American Medical Association's code of ethics for physicians). Among the oldest of these and the best known is the ancient Hippocratic oath, versions of which have been taken by many medical school classes at graduation.

The field of medical ethics (biomedical ethics, bioethics) has greatly expanded in the context of many new and difficult issues, such as those related to death and dying and the conflicts between humanism and technology, which have confronted professionals, patients, and families. Many of these matters have come to be adjudicated in the courts and can be viewed as ethical–legal issues. Among the many ethical issues in health and medical care, several have drawn particular attention.

Death and Dying ("Death with Dignity")

There has been great interest in humanizing the care of dying patients, particularly those with terminal cancer. A large body of medical and ethical (and legal) literature has developed on the subject.

One reflection of this concern is the development of the *hospice* movement. (See page 53.)

A closely related issue is that of the prolongation of the life of the hopelessly ill by technological means, including life support apparatus such as the respirator. The issue of removing unconscious and irreversible brain damaged patients from such equipment ("pulling the plug") has come before the courts in a number of widely publicized cases.

Among the best known cases involving technological life support is that of *Karen Ann Quinlan*, which was decided in the state of New Jersey in 1976.[8] This young woman was in an irreversible coma and being maintained on a respirator. Her parents requested that this support be terminated, but the attending physician declined, whereupon her father asked the court to appoint him guardian for the purpose of discontinuing this "extraordinary" means of care. The New Jersey Supreme Court ultimately held that Mr. Quinlan as guardian might seek the withdrawal of the life support system with the concurrence of attending physicians in consultation with a hospital "ethics" committee, without civil or criminal liability for physicians or others. In essence, the decision to continue life sustaining apparatus was left to the family and physicians.

On the other hand, in the *Saikewicz decision*[9] of the Massachusetts Supreme Court has been interpreted as holding that the question of withholding life extending measures in hopelessly ill, incompetent persons should be left to the courts and not others. (The patient in question was a very mentally retarded man terminally ill with leukemia and the treatment at issue was a course of chemotherapy.) The same court later tried to clarify its position in the *Spring decision*[10] involving a markedly senile man who required renal dialysis treatments, although the exact circumstances under which the courts would have to be involved remained unclear.

Physicians have often refrained from taking measures to prolong the life of the hopelessly ill and many people have argued that this should remain a medical and ethical decision. However these matters are coming to the courts with increasing frequency.

---

8. *In re Quinlan*, 355 A.2nd 647 (1976).

9. *Superintendant of Belchertown State School* v. *Saikewicz*, Mass 370 N.E. 2d 647 (1976).

10. *In re Spring*, 405 N.E.2d 115 (1980).

A related issue is that of supporting the life of newborn infants who have serious birth defects and who, if they survive, will be left with extensive physical or mental handicaps. This has been much debated as technological advances permit the survival of such infants who otherwise would have died naturally. These decisions have generally been made by physicians and parents but the issues are very controversial and instances of disagreement between parents and physicians in individual cases are not uncommon.[11]

The Living Will.   It is generally held that competent adults have the right to refuse treatment, including life prolonging treatment. This right to "die naturally" has been much discussed. A *living will* is an explicit statement, oral or written, by a competent adult that makes it clear that he or she does not wish life sustaining measures to be used in the event of hopeless illness. A number of states have passed laws explicitly recognizing such requests. These have been termed "death with dignity," "right to die," and "natural death" laws. The first such law enacted was the 1976 California *Natural Death Act*, which recognized "the right of an adult person to make a written directive instructing his physician to withhold or withdraw life sustaining procedures in the event of terminal condition."

Euthanasia.[12]   Euthanasia is the inducing or permitting of a painless death where ethically justified, such as in cases of particularly painful terminal illness. The withholding of treatment that would prolong life is called *passive, negative,* or *indirect* euthanasia. A positive action to hasten death is called *active, positive,* or *direct* euthanasia. (Some such actions have been called "mercy killings.") Passive euthanasia, particularly that involving the withholding of "extraordinary" means of treatment, has been widely condoned. Active euthanasia, though advocated by some, is not generally condoned and can be criminally prosecuted.

11. See, for example, "On the Death of a Baby" by Robert and Peggy Stinson. *The Atlantic Monthly*, July 1979.

12. From the Greek *eu* (good) and *thanatos* (death).

Human Experimentation

The ethics of human experimentation has been the subject of much discussion and debate, particularly since the increasing recognition of ethical problems related to biomedical research and the development of new diagnostic and therapeutic techniques and drugs. A number of past research programs, including some carried out in closed institutions such as prisons and institutions for the mentally retarded, have come under criticism. It is now widely accepted that, in general, human subjects should participate in research experiments with informed consent and in the case of patients (as distinct from healthy volunteers), there should be some potential benefit to the individual participating. Ethical concerns have led to the widespread establishment of *institutional review boards* to review and approve research proposals that involve human subjects. Such review mechanisms are required for research funded by the federal government.

Patients' Rights

The rights of patients have been the subject of concern by consumer and advocacy groups and ethicists. Informed consent, explanations of diagnoses and treatment, and access to medical records are among the matters frequently addressed. A number of hospitals have formalized a "bill of rights" for patients and some state legislatures have made patients' rights in hospitals and nursing homes a matter of statutory law.

Abortion

Abortion is an example of an action whose legality has been affirmed (by the Supreme Court in 1973) but that has remained a hotly debated ethical and moral issue. The continuing debate has led to some successful efforts to constrain its practice, such as by restricting the use of public funds to pay for the procedure.[13]

---

13. Notably, the Hyde Amendment to recent Congressional appropriations bills forbidding federal Medicaid funding of abortions.

Organizations and Commissions

Two particularly well-known organizations active in the field of medical ethics are the *Institute of Society, Ethics and the Life Sciences*, Hastings-on-Hudson, New York, also known as the *Hastings Center*; and the *Kennedy Institute for the Study of Human Reproduction and Bioethics*, Georgetown University, Washington, D.C.

The *National Commission for the Protection of Human Subjects of Biomedical and Behavioral Research*, established by Congress in 1974 (PL 93-348), carried out studies and made various recommendations related to human research subjects. Its work is being continued, with a broader mandate, by the *President's Commission for the Study of Ethical Problems in Medicine and Biomedical and Behavioral Research*, established by Congress in 1978 (PL 95-622). Ethical issues being addressed include those related to allocation of health resources and access to care.

SELECTED READINGS

The Law of Hospital and Health Care Administration, Arthur Southwick (Ann Arbor: Health Administration Press, 1978).

Law, Medicine, and Forensic Science, 3rd ed., William J. Curran and E. Donald Shapiro (Boston: Little, Brown and Company, 1982).

The Rights of Hospital Patients (an American Civil Liberties Union Handbook), George J. Annas (New York: Avon Books, 1975).

The Rights of Doctors, Nurses and Allied Health Professionals: A Health Law Primer (an American Civil Liberties Union Handbook), George J. Annas, Leonard H. Glantz, and Barbara F. Katz [New York: Avon Books (paperback) Cambridge, Massachusetts: Ballinger Publishing Company, 1981 (cloth)].

On Human Care and Introduction to Ethics, Arthur Dyck (Nashville, Tennessee: Abington Press, 1977).

Principles of Biomedical Ethics, Tom L. Beauchamp and James F. Childress (New York: Oxford University Press, 1979).

APPENDICES

SELECTED HISTORICAL LANDMARKS[1]

1620   The physician, Samuel Fuller, arrives with the Pilgrims on the Mayflower at Plymouth, Massachusetts.

1639   Virginia passed the first law regulating medical practice.

1721   Smallpox inoculation used in Boston and demonstrated effective.

1756   Pennsylvania Hospital in Philadelphia founded. The oldest U.S. hospital in existence.

1765   The first medical school (Medical School of the College of Philadelphia).

1790s   Local boards of health organized in Baltimore, Boston, Philadelphia, and New York City.

1798   U.S. Public Health Service established by Congress, then called the Marine Hospital Service.

1800   First U.S. use of smallpox vaccination by Dr. Benjamin Waterhouse.

1812   Start of the original version of the *New England Journal of Medicine* now the oldest U.S. medical journal.

---

1. Also see Appendix C, Chronological List of Laws.

1842   First use of ether anesthesia in Georgia by Dr. Crawford Long.

1846   First public demonstration of ether anesthesia—Boston, Massachusetts.

1847   American Medical Association founded.

1850   Lemuel Shattuck's *Report of the Sanitary Commission of Massachusetts* proposes important public health reforms.

1855   Louisiana establishes the first State Health Department.

1872   American Public Health Association formed.

1873   First nursing schools based on Florence Nightingale's principles.

1874   Dr. A.T. Still defines osteopathic medicine.

1887   First national census of hospitals. There were 187 of them. By 1915 there are over 5,000 hospitals.
Charles Mayo and his sons William and Charles establish a practice in Rochester, Minnesota. This evolved into the Mayo Clinic, the first large medical group practice.

1896   Roentgen's x-ray paper arrives in the United States and the technique is quickly applied in several places.

1878   Founding of the American Hospital Association.

1906   Pure Food and Drug Act passed. This becomes the basis for the federal regulation of foods and drugs.

1910   Abraham Flexner's Report on *Medical Education in the United States and Canada*, Carnegie Foundation.

1910   First university-based school of nursing (University of Minnesota).

1912   Children's Bureau created as part of the Department of Labor of the Federal Government.

1913   Founding of the American College of Surgeons.

1917   American Board of Ophthalmology formed. The first medical specialty board.

1929   Blue Cross concept starts at Baylor University.

1937   The National Cancer Act of 1937 provides for the establishment of the National Cancer Institute.

1942   Kaiser Permanente Health Plan formed.

1946   Hill Burton hospital planning and construction legislation.

1951   The Joint Commission on Accreditation of Hospitals formed, taking over accreditation activities carried out by the American College of Surgeons since 1918.

1955   The high point in the total number of mental patients in U.S. hospitals. Effective antipsychotic drugs and the community mental health movement reduced this number.

1965   Medicare and Medicaid legislation passed.

In the last thirty years changes in U.S. health services have resulted largely from advances in biomedical research and technology and from federal government legislation.

ALPHABET SOUP[1]

A	AABB	American Association of Blood Banks
	AAMC	Association of American Medical Colleges
	ABC	American Blood Commission
	ACS	American College of Surgeons
	ACGME	Accreditation Council for Graduate Medical Education
	ADA	American Dental Association
		American Dietetic Association
	ADAMHA	Alcohol Drug Abuse and Mental Health Administration
	AFDC	Aid to Families with Dependent Children
	AGPA	American Group Practice Association
	AHA	American Hospital Association
	AHEC	Area Health Education Center
	ALOS	Average Length of Stay
	AMA	American Medical Association
	AMHT	Automated Multi-Phasic Health Testing
	ANA	American Nurses' Association
	AOA	American Osteopathic Association
	APA	American Podiatry Association
		American Psychological Association

1. This selected list contains abbreviations noted in the text.

	APhA	American Pharmaceutical Association
	APHA	American Public Health Association
	ART	Accredited Record Technician
	ASCP	American Society of Clinical Pathologists
	ASTHO	Association of State and Territorial Health Officials
	AUPHA	Association of University Programs in Health Administration
B	BC	Blue Cross
	BCA	Blue Cross Association
	BS	Blue Shield
	BX	Blue Cross
C	CAHEA	Committee on Allied Health Education and Accreditation
	CCU	Coronary Care Unit
	CDC	Centers for Disease Control
	CEO	Chief Executive Officer
	CEU	Continuing Education Unit
	CHAMPUS	Civilian Health and Medical Program of the Uniformed Services
	CHAMPVA	Civilian Health and Medical Program of the Veterans Administration
	CLA	Certified Laboratory Technician
	CME	Continuing Medical Education
	CMHC	Community Mental Health Center
	CON	Certificate of Need
	CPC	Clinico-Pathological Conference
	CPHA	Commission on Professional and Hospital Activities
	CT	Computed Tomography
	CT (ASCP)	Registered Cytotechnologist
	C&Y	Children and Youth Project
D	DAT	Dental Aptitude Test
	DC	Doctor of Chiropractic
	DDS	Doctor of Dental Surgery
	DEA	Drug Enforcement Administration
	DMD	Doctor of Dental Medicine
	DO	Doctor of Osteopathy

	DOD	Department of Defense
	DON	Determination of Need
	DRG	Diagnosis Related Groups
	DSC	Doctor of Surgical Chiropody
	DVM	Doctor of Veterinary Medicine
E	ECF	Extended Care Facility
	ECFMG	Educational Commission for Foreign Medical Graduates
	ED	Emergency Department
	EDDA	Expanded Duty Dental Assistant
	EEG	Electroencephalograph
	EKG (ECG)	Electrocardiograph
	EMCRO	Experimental Medical Review Organization
	EMT	Emergency Medical Technician
	EPA	Environmental Protection Agency
	EPSDT	Early and Periodic Screening, Diagnosis and Treatment
	ER	Emergency Room
	ESRD	End-Stage Renal Disease Program
	EW	Emergency Ward
F	FDA	Food and Drug Administration
	FEHBP	Federal Employees Health Benefits Program
	FLEX	Federation Licensing Examination
	FMC	Foundation for Medical Care
	FMG	Foreign Medical Graduate
	FP	Family Practitioner
	FTC	Federal Trade Commission
	FY	Fiscal Year
G	GME	Graduate Medical Education
	GP	General Practitioner
H	HCFA	Health Care Financing Administration
	HEW	Department of Health, Education and Welfare
	HHS	Department of Health and Human Services
	HIAA	Health Insurance Association of America
	HIP	Health Insurance Plan of Greater New York
	HMO	Health Maintenance Organization
	HRA	Health Resources Administration

	HSA	Health Services Administration
		Health Systems Agency
	HT (ASCP)	Histologic Technician
	HUD	Department of Housing and Urban Development
	HUP	Hospital Utilization Project of Pennsylvania
I	ICF	Intermediate Care Facility
	ICU	Intensive Care Unit
	IOM	Institute of Medicine
	IPA	Individual Practice Association
J	JCAH	Joint Commission on Accreditation of Hospitals
L	LCME	Liaison Committee on Medical Education
	LOS	Length of Stay
	LPN	Licensed Practical Nurse
	LVN	Licensed Vocational Nurse
M	MAP	Medical Audit Program
	MCAT	Medical College Admission Test
	MCH	Maternal and Child Health
	MD	Doctor of Medicine
	MEDLARS	Medical Literature and Analysis Retrieval System
	MIC	Maternal and Infant Care Project
	MICU	Mobile Intensive Care Unit
	MPH	Master of Public Health
	MSW	Master of Social Work
	MT (ASCP)	Medical Technologist
N	NABSP	National Association of Blue Shield Plans
	NASW	National Association of Social Workers
	NBME	National Board of Medical Examiners
	NCHCT	National Center for Health Care Technology
	NCHS	National Center for Health Statistics
	NCHSR	National Center for Health Services Research
	NDA	New Drug Application
	NF	National Formulary
	NHSC	National Health Service Corps
	NIH	National Institutes of Health
	NIMH	National Institute of Mental Health
	NIOSH	National Institute of Occupational Safety and Health

	NLN	National League for Nursing
	NLRB	National Labor Relations Board
	NP	Nurse Practitioner
	NRMP	National Resident Matching Program
O	OASDI	Old Age, Survivors and Disability Insurance (Social Security)
	OD	Doctor of Optometry
	OEO	Office of Economic Opportunity
	OMB	Office of Management and Budget
	OPD	Outpatient Department
	OR	Operating Room
	OSHA	Occupational Safety and Health Administration
	OTA	Office of Technology Assessment, U.S. Congress
	OTC	Over the Counter Drugs
	OTR	Registered Occupational Therapist
P	PA	Physician's Assistant
	PAS	Professional Activity Study
	PDR	Physicians' Desk Reference
	PGP	Prepaid Group Practice
	PGY	Post Graduate Year
	PHS	Public Health Service (also USPHS)
	PMA	Pharmaceutical Manufacturers' Association
	Pod.D.	Doctor of Podiatry
	POMR	Problem Oriented Medical Record
	PPC	Progressive Patient Care
	PSRO	Professional Standards Review Organization
	PT	Physical Therapist, Physical Therapy
Q	QAP	Quality Assurance Program
R	RCC	Ratio of Costs to Charges
	RCT	Randomized Control or Clinical Trial
	RFP	Request for Proposal
	RN	Registered Nurse
	RPh	Registered Pharmacist
	RRA	Registered Record Administrator
	RVS	Relative Value Scale
S	SHCC	Statewide Health Coordinating Council
	SHPDA	State Health Planning and Development Agency

	SMA	Sequential Multiple Analyzer
	SMSA	Standard Metropolitan Statistical Area
	SNF	Skilled Nursing Facility
	SSA	Social Security Administration
	SSI	Supplemental Security Income
T	Title XVIII,	
	XIX	Sections of Social Security Act (Medicare and Medicaid)
U	UCR	Usual, Customary, and Reasonable
	UR	Utilization Review
	USAN	United States Adopted Names Council
	USP	United States Pharmacopeia
	USPHS	United States Public Health Service
V	VA	Veterans Administration
	VISTA	Volunteers in Service to America
	VMD	Doctor of Veterinary Medicine
	VNA	Visiting Nurse Association

CHRONOLOGICAL LIST OF LAWS[1]

1906   Pure Food and Drug Act PL 59–384

1908   Federal Employees Compensation Act PL 60–176

1917   Vocational Education Act PL 64–347

1920   Vocational Rehabilitation Act PL 66–236

1921   Maternity and Infancy Act PL 67–97

1935   *Social Security Act PL 74–271

1943   Vocational Rehabilitation Amendments of 1943
        PL 78–113
        Emergency Maternal and Infant Care Act PL 78–156

1944   *Public Health Service Act PL 78–410

1946   *National Mental Health Act PL 79–487
        *Hospital Survey and Construction Act PL 79–725
        *Vocational Education Act of 1946 PL 79–586

1949   *Hospital Survey and Construction Amendments of 1949
        PL 81–380

---

1. Major laws described or referred to in this book.
*Official short title.

1954   *Medical Facilities Survey and Construction Act of 1954
        PL 83-482
        *Dependents Medical Care Act PL 83-569

1956   *Health Research Facilities Act of 1956 PL 84-835
        *Health Amendments Act of 1956 PL 84-911
        *National Health Survey Act PL 84-652

1958   Grants-in-aid to Schools of Public Health PL 85-544

1959   *Federal Employees Health Benefits Act of 1959
        PL 86-352

1960   *Social Security Amendments of 1960 PL 86-778
        Graduate Training in Public Health PL 86-720

1961   *Community Health Services and Facilities Act of 1961
        PL 87-395

1962   Health Services for Agricultural Migratory Workers
        PL 87-692

1963   *Health Professions Educational Assistance Act of 1963
        PL 88-129
        *Maternal and Child Health and Mental Retardation
        Planning Amendments of 1963 PL 88-156
        *Mental Retardation Facilities and Community Mental
        Health Centers Construction Act of 1963 PL 88-164

1964   *Hospital and Medical Facilities Amendments of 1964
        PL 88-443
        *Economic Opportunity Act of 1964 PL 88-452
        *Graduate Public Health Training Amendments of 1964
        PL 88-497
        *Nurse Training Act PL 88-581

1965   *Appalachian Redevelopment Act of 1965 PL 89-4
        *Social Security Amendments of 1965 PL 89-97
        *Mental Retardation Facilities and Community Mental
        Health Centers Construction Act Amendments of 1965
        PL 89-105
        *Heart Disease, Cancer and Stroke Amendments of 1965
        PL 89-239

*Official short title.

*Health Professions Educational Assistance Amendments of 1965 PL 89-290

1966 *Comprehensive Health Planning and Public Health Service Amendments of 1966 PL 89-749
*Allied Health Professions Personnel Training Act of 1966 PL 89-751

1967 *Mental Health Amendments of 1967 PL 90-31
*Mental Retardation Amendments of 1967 PL 90-170
*Partnership for Health Amendments PL 90-174
*Social Security Amendments of 1967 PL 90-248

1968 *Health Manpower Act of 1968 PL 90-490
Public Health Service Amendments of 1968 PL 90-574

1969 *Federal Coal Mine Health and Safety Act of 1969 PL 91-173

1970 *Community Mental Health Centers Amendments of 1970 PL 91-211
*Medical Facilities Construction and Modernization Amendments of 1970 PL 91-296
*Communicable Disease Control Amendments of 1970 PL 91-464
*Comprehensive Drug Abuse Prevention and Control Act of 1970 PL 91-513
Public Health Service Amendments PL 91-515
*Health Training Improvement Act of 1970 PL 91-519
*Occupational Safety and Health Act of 1970 PL 91-596
*Family Planning Services and Population Research Act of 1970 PL 91-572
*Comprehensive Alcohol Abuse and Alcoholism Prevention, Treatment, and Rehabilitation Act of 1970 PL 91-616
*Emergency Health Personnel Act of 1970 PL 91-623
*Lead-Based Paint Poisoning Prevention Act PL 91-695

1971 *Nurse Training Act of 1971 PL 92-158
*Comprehensive Health Manpower Training Act of 1971 PL 92-157
*National Cancer Act of 1971 PL 92-218
Social Security Amendments PL 92-223

*Official short title.

1972   *National Sickle Cell Anemia Control Act PL 92-294
        *Communicable Disease Control Amendments of 1972
          PL 92-449
        *Social Security Amendments of 1972 PL 92-603
        *National Cooley's Anemia Control Act PL 92-714
        *Uniformed Services Health Professions Revitalization Act
          of 1972 PL 92-426
        *State and Local Fiscal Assistance Act of 1972 PL 92-512
        *Consumer Product Safety Act PL 92-573

1973   *Health Programs Extension Act of 1973 PL 93-45
        *Emergency Medical Services Systems Act PL 93-154
        *Health Maintenance Organization Act of 1973 PL 93-222

1974   *Sudden Infant Death Syndrome Act of 1974 PL 93-270
        *Congressional Budget and Impoundment Control Act of
          1974 PL 93-344
        Nonprofit Hospital Amendments (National Labor Rela-
          tions Act) PL 93-360
        *Rehabilitation Act Amendments of 1974 PL 93-516
        *National Health Planning and Resources Development Act
          of 1974 PL 93-641
        *Headstart, Economic Opportunity and Community Partner-
          ship Act of 1974 PL 93-644
        *Social Services Amendments of 1974 PL 93-647

1975   Public Health and Community Mental Health Amend-
          ments PL 94-63
        *Developmentally Disabled Assistance and Bill of Rights
          Act PL 94-103

1976   *Medical Devices Amendments of 1976 PL 94-295
        *National Consumer Health Information and Health Promo-
          tion Act of 1976 PL 94-317
        *Health Maintenance Organization Amendments of 1976
          PL 94-460
        *Health Professions Educational Assistance Act of 1976
          PL 94-484

* Official short title

1977   *Medicare–Medicaid Antifraud and Abuse Amendments PL 95–142
Rural Health Clinic Services Amendments (Medicare) PL 95–210

1978   Medicare End-Stage Renal Disease Amendments PL 95–292
Health Maintenance Organization Amendments of 1978 PL 95–559

1979   Health Planning and Resources Development Amendments of 1979 PL 96–79

1980   *Medicare and Medicaid Amendments of 1980 (Title IX, Omnibus Reconciliation Act of 1980) PL 96–499
*Mental Health Systems Act PL 96–398

1981   Omnibus Budget Reconciliation Act of 1981 PL 97–35

*Official short title

SUMMARY OF THE SOCIAL SECURITY ACT (1935)

Title I *Grants to the States for Old Age Assistance*

Provided grants to the states for financial assistance to needy aged.

Title II *Federal Old Age Benefits*

Set up the federal "Social Security" program of old age benefits based on wages earned before age sixty-five.[1]

Title III *Grants to the States for Unemployment Compensation Administration*

Provided federal payment for the administrative expenses of state programs for unemployment compensation.

Title IV *Grants to the States for Aid to Dependent Children*

Provided for grants to the states for financial aid for needy dependent children.[2]

1. There were many exclusions in the original act, including domestic and agricultural labor, employees of government and nonprofit agencies, and the self-employed. Coverage since has been gradually extended and at present includes more than 90 percent of working people. (Railway workers are similarly covered under the Railroad Retirement Act; federal employees also have a separate program.)

2. Children under age sixteen deprived of parental support through death, absence or incapacity of a parent, and living with relatives. Payments are now authorized for children up to age twenty-one providing they are in school.

Title V   *Grants to the States for Maternal and Child Welfare*

Provided grants to the states for maternal and child health and child welfare services, and services to crippled children. Administration of the program was assigned to the Children's Bureau.[3] (Also extended vocational rehabilitation programs previously authorized under other legislation.)

Title VI   *Public Health Work*

Provided grants to the states for state and local public health services and additional funds for programs of the Public Health Service.

Title VII   *Social Security Board*

Established the Social Security Board to administer the programs authorized under the act (with the exception of those in Titles V and VI), and to study and make recommendations regarding economic security and social insurance.

Title VIII *Taxes with Respect to Employment*

Levied a payroll tax on employees eligible for the federal old age benefits program, and a tax in equal amount on their employers.

Title IX   *Tax on Employers of Eight or More*

Levied an additional tax on employers that could be credited against contributions to state unemployment funds. Its purpose was to encourage the establishment of such funds by the states.

Title X   *Grants to the States for Aid to the Blind*

Provided grants to the states for financial assistance to needy blind persons.

Title XI   *General Provisions*

Contained general definitions and administrative regulations.

---

3. This title in effect re-established and expanded the program of assistance for maternal and child health programs previously authorized under the federal Maternity and Infancy Act (1921–29), which was the first federal grant-in-aid program for direct health services.

SOCIAL SECURITY AMENDMENTS OF 1965*

Title XVIII, Health Insurance for the Aged (Medicare)

Part A: Hospital Insurance Benefits. This insurance program provides basic protection against the costs of hospital and related post-hospital services. Benefits consist of entitlement to have payment made for:

- *Inpatient hospital* services up to 90 days during any spell of illness and psychiatric inpatient services up to 190 days in a lifetime.
- Posthospital *extended care* services up to 100 days during any spell of illness.
- Posthospital *home health* services up to 100 visits in a one-year period.
- Hospital outpatient diagnostic services.

The amount payable for these services (except home health) is subject to deductible and coinsurance payments by the beneficiary as follows:

- *Inpatient*: $40 deductible until January 1, 1969, thereafter to be increased according to the increase in average per diem rates for

---

*Summary.

in-hospital services;[1] coinsurance, equal to one-fourth the deductible for each day after the sixtieth hospital day.

- *Extended care*: no deductible; coinsurance, equal to one-eighth the inpatient hospital deductible for each day after the twentieth day.
- *Home health services*: no deductible or coinsurance.
- *Outpatient*: for services provided in a twenty-day period by one hospital, deductible is equal to one-half the inpatient deductible; coinsurance is equal to 20 percent of the remaining amount payable.

The conditions for payment to providers of service include:

- Written request by beneficiary (except where found impracticable by the Secretary).
- *Certification* by a physician of the necessity for the services, and periodic recertification where applicable, beginning no later than the twentieth day.
- For psychiatric hospital services, certification that such treatment can reasonably be expected to improve the condition for which treatment is necessary.
- For tuberculosis hospital services, certification that treatment can reasonably be expected to improve the condition or render it noncommunicable.
- For posthospital extended care services, certification of the need for skilled nursing care for condition for which the preceding inpatient services were received.
- For posthospital home health services, certification that services are required because the individual is confined to his or her home and needs skilled nursing care, or physical or speech therapy for conditions for which he or she was receiving inpatient hospital services.

The amount paid to any provider of services must be the *reasonable cost* of such services.

---

1. The deductible was considered to represent roughly the cost of the first hospital day.

Payment may be made for emergency services provided by a non-participating hospital including, under limited conditions, hospitals outside the United States.

Groups of associations of providers of services may elect to have payments made through a public or private agency or organization.[2] The Secretary is authorized to make agreements with such designated organizations by which they will determine the payments to be made for services and will make such payments. These agencies may be required to:

- Provide consultation to providers for their establishment of necessary fiscal records and the meeting of other qualifications.
- Serve as a center for communication of information between the Secretary and the providers.
- Make necessary audits of records of providers.

The nomination of an agency or organization, however, is not binding on individual members of the nominating association or group.

A *Federal Hospital Insurance Trust Fund* is established for payments under Part A. The trust fund is to be financed by an earnings tax paid by employees, employers, and the self-employed.

Part B: Supplementary Medical Insurance Benefits. This is a voluntary insurance program financed from premium payments by enrollees and contributions from federal funds. Benefits consist of entitlement to have payment made for:

- Home health services up to 100 visits in a year.
- Medical and other health services:
    a. physicians' services
    b. services and supplies incidental to a physician's professional services
    c. diagnostic x-ray, laboratory, and other tests
    d. radiotherapy
    e. surgical dressings, splints, casts

2. These nonfederal agencies that deal directly with the providers of services are known as *fiscal intermediaries*.

   f. rental of durable medical equipment used in the home

   g. ambulance service (with limitations)

   h. prosthetic devices (except dental) and braces

Independent laboratories providing services under this program must be approved by the Secretary.

Payments for physicians' services are to be 80 percent of reasonable charges, and may be made to the beneficiary or on his or her behalf. (An organization providing services on a prepayment basis may be paid 80 percent of reasonable costs.)

Payments for other medical and health services are to be 80 percent of *reasonable costs.*

Medical and other health services under this part are subject to a $50 deductible in each calendar year. (Expenses incurred for hospital outpatient diagnostic services under Part A may be counted toward the deductible.)

With regard to out of hospital psychiatric services, there shall be considered as incurred expense in any year, no more than $250 after the deductible.

The conditions for payment to providers of services include:

- Written *request by beneficiary*, unless impracticable.

- In the case of *home health* services, *certification by a physician* that the individual is confined to his or her home and needs skilled nursing care or physical or speech therapy and that services are furnished while the individual is under the care of a physician.

- In the case of other medical or health services, certification by a physician, that these were medically required.

Provision is made for general and individual *enrollment periods.*

The *initial monthly premium is set at $3.* Beginning in 1968, the monthly premium shall be determined every two years on the basis of the benefit and administrative costs of the program.

For persons receiving monthly Social Security benefits, premiums will be deducted from these payments.

A *Federal Supplementary Insurance Trust Fund* is established for payments under Part B.

The Surgeon General is authorized to enter into contracts with (health insurance) carriers for administration of these benefits.

The carriers will:

- Determine rates and amounts of payments required, disburse and account for funds, and make necessary audits of records of providers of services.

- Assist in development of procedures relating to utilization practices and determine compliance with requirements for utilization review.

- Serve as a channel for communication of information relating to the administration of this program.

- Assure that payments are made for reasonable costs, and for charges that are reasonable and not higher than the charges applicable for comparable services to the policyholders and subscribers of the carrier. Payments for charges may be made on the basis of a receipted bill or on the basis of an *assignment*. In the latter case the reasonable charge will be the full charge for the services.

In determining the reasonable charge for services there shall be taken into consideration the *customary charges* for similar services generally made by physicians or other persons furnishing such services, as well as the *prevailing* charges in the locality.

The Surgeon General, at the request of a state, will enter into an agreement whereby eligible individuals in the federally aided *public assistance categories* will be enrolled in Part B with the monthly premium to be paid by the state.

A government contribution will be made from the Treasury equal to the *aggregate premiums* payable under this part.[3]

Part C: Miscellaneous Provisions. Definitions[4] (for purposes of Title XVIII) include:

- Spell of Illness—a period beginning with the first day on which an individual is furnished inpatient hospital services or extended care services and ending with the close of the first period of sixty consecutive days thereafter on each of which he or she is neither an inpatient of a hospital or an extended care facility.

---

3. That is, half the costs of Part B will be paid from general revenues.
4. Abbreviated.

- Inpatient Hospital Service—(1) bed and board; (2) such nursing services, use of hospital facilities, medical social services, and such drugs, biological supplies, appliances, and equipment, for use in the hospital, as are ordinarily furnished to inpatients by a hospital.

  Excluded are physicians' services (except interns and residents under a training program) and the services of *private duty nurses.*

- Hospital—an institution that:
  a. Is primarily engaged in providing by or under the supervision of physicians, to inpatients, services for diagnosis, treatment, care, or rehabilitation.
  b. Maintains clinical records on all patients.
  c. Has bylaws in effect with respect to its staff of physicians.
  d. Has a requirement that every patient must be under the care of a physician.
  e. Provides twenty-four hour nursing service rendered or supervised by a registered professional nurse.
  f. Has in effect a hospital *utilization review plan.*
  g. If in any state whose laws provide for licensing of hospitals, is so licensed or meets the standards for licensure.
  h. Meets such other requirements as the Secretary finds necessary in the interest of the health and safety of hospitalized individuals except that such requirements may not be higher than the comparable requirements of the Joint Commission on Accreditation of Hospitals.

- Extended Care Facility—an institution (or distinct part of an institution) that has in effect a *transfer agreement* with one or more participating hospitals and that:
  a. Is primarily engaged in providing to inpatients *skilled nursing care* or *rehabilitation* services.
  b. Has policies that are developed with the advice of a group of professional personnel, and has a physician, a registered professional nurse or a medical staff responsible for the execution of such policies.
  c. Requires that every patient be under the supervision of a physician and provides for having a physician available in case of emergency.
  d. Maintains clinical records on all patients.

e. Provides twenty-four nursing service sufficient to meet nursing needs in accordance with the policies developed and has at least one registered nurse employed full time.
f. Provides appropriate methods and procedures for the dispensing and administering of drugs and biologicals.
g. Has a *utilization review plan.*
h. If in any state with laws providing for licensing of such institutions, is so licensed or meets the licensure standards.
i. Meets such other conditions relating to the health and safety of its patients as the Secretary may find necessary.

- Utilization Review—a utilization review plan of a hospital or extended care facility is considered sufficient if it is applicable to services to individuals entitled to insurance benefits under this title. It is to provide:

a. For review, on a sample or other basis, of admissions, *duration of stay* and professional services with respect to *medical necessity* and to promote the most efficient use of facilities and services.
b. For review to be made by a staff committee of two or more physicians, with or without other professional personnel or a similar group established by the local medical society and some or all of the hospitals and extended care facilities in the locality.
c. For review of cases of *extended duration.*
d. For prompt notification to the institution, the individual, and his or her physician of any finding (made after opportunity for consultation with such physician) that further stay in the institution is not medically necessary).

- Home Health Agency—an agency or organization that:

a. Is primarily engaged in providing skilled nursing services and other therapeutic services.
b. Has policies established by a group of professional personnel including one or more physicians and one or more registered professional nurses, and provides for supervision of such services by a physician or a registered professional nurse.
c. Maintains clinical records on all patients.
d. If in any state providing for the licensing of organizations of this nature, is so licensed or meets the licensure standards.

e. Meets such other conditions of participation as the Secretary may find necessary in the interest of individuals furnished services.

- Home Health Services—the following items and services furnished to an individual under the care of a physician by a home health agency on a visiting basis in an individual's home:
  a. Nursing care provided by or under the supervision of a registered professional nurse.
  b. Physical, occupational, or speech therapy.
  c. Medical *social services*.
  d. Home health aid services.
  e. Medical supplies and use of medical appliances.
  f. Any of the foregoing provided on an outpatient basis at a hospital, extended care facility, or rehabilitation center that involves the use of equipment that cannot be made readily available in the home.

- Posthospital Extended Care Services—extended care service furnished an individual after transfer from a hospital in which he or she was an inpatient for not less than three consecutive days; admission to the extended care facility to be not more than fourteen days after discharge from such hospital.

- Posthospital Home Health Services—home health services furnished an individual within one year after his or her most recent discharge from a hospital of which he or she was an inpatient for not less than three consecutive days, or from an extended care facility (in which he or she was an inpatient under Part A). In either case, the plan for home health services is to be established within fourteen days after such discharge.

- Physician—a licensed doctor of medicine, osteopathy, or dentistry.

- Provider of Services—a hospital, extended care facility, or home health agency.

Payment is to be made for the reasonable cost of *semiprivate* accommodations: two bed, three bed, or four bed. Payment may exceed semiprivate cost only if more expensive accommodations are required for medical reasons. If accommodations furnished are less expensive than semiprivate, payment will be minus the difference.

Excluded from coverage are (among others):

- Services that are not provided within the United States (except emergency services).
- Personal comfort items.
- Routine physical checkups; eyeglasses or related eye examinations; hearing aids or related examinations; immunizations.
- Orthopedic shoes or other supportive devices for the feet.
- Custodial care.
- Cosmetic surgery except as required for repair of accidental injury or improvement of functioning of a malformed body member.
- Care, treatment, filling, removal, or replacement of teeth.
- Services provided under a workmen's compensation law.

In developing conditions of participation for providers of services the Secretary shall consult with the Health Insurance Benefits Advisory Council, appropriate state agencies, recognized national listing or accrediting bodies and may consult with appropriate local agencies.

The Secretary shall make an agreement with any state willing and able to do so whereby an appropriate state or local agency may determine whether an institution is a hospital or extended care facility, or an agency is a home health agency (as these terms are defined) or whether a laboratory meets the stated requirements. The Secretary may also agree to utilize the services of such agencies to provide consultation to institutions or agencies to assist them to establish and maintain fiscal records or otherwise to qualify as providers of services, including the establishment of utilization review procedures. The requirements for a participating hospital shall be deemed to have been met if an institution is accredited as a hospital by the *Joint Commission on Accreditation of Hospitals* (provided that utilization review procedures are also established).[5]

A *Health Insurance Benefits Advisory Council* of sixteen members is established to advise the Secretary on general policy in the administration of this Title and in the formulation of regulations. Members

---

5. Accreditation by the American Osteopathic Association or other national accredita body may also be accepted.

to include persons in fields related to hospital, medical, and other health activities and at least one person representing the general public.

A *National Medical Review Committee* of nine members is established to include individuals who are representative of organizations and associations of professional personnel in the field of medicine, other individuals from medicine or related fields, and at least one member representative of the general public; a majority of the members to be physicians. The function of the Committee is to study the utilization of hospital and other medical care and services provided under this Title with a view to recommending any changes that may seem desirable in the way in which such services are utilized and in the administration of the programs established by this Title.

The Secretary shall prescribe such regulations as may be necessary to carry out the administration of this program.

Eligibility. Persons eligible are those who have attained the age of 65 and are entitled to monthly Social Security or railroad retirement benefits. Other persons are eligible under transitional provisions, provided they attain age 65 before 1968 and are resident citizens of the United States or have been permanent resident aliens for at least five years. Excluded are those eligible for the Federal Employee Health Benefits Program and those convicted of specific crimes against national security.

Title XIX, Grants to the States for Medical Assistance Programs (Medicaid)

> For the purpose of enabling each state to furnish medical assistance on behalf of families with dependent children and of aged, blind, or permanently and totally disabled individuals whose income and resources are insufficient to meet the costs of necessary medical services ..."

This Title establishes a single new program of medical assistance for persons receiving federally aided public assistance[6] and extends eligibility to comparable groups of *medically indigent persons*, that is, needy families with dependent children, and blind, disabled, or

6. Persons eligible for Aid to Families with Dependent Children, Old Age Assistance, Aid to the Blind, and Aid to the Permanently and Totally Disabled.

elderly persons who are not on welfare. All *needy children* (under 21) are also made eligible.

The federal share of the program's costs is 50 to 83 percent, according to a state's per capita income.

Participation in the new medical assistance program is optional for the states, who can elect to continue (until January 1970) under the old medical provisions of the public assistance titles. After January 1970 federal payments for medical care of the medically indigent aged (Kerr–Mills program) will be made only under the new program, which would now have to include the other groups as well. A state not starting the new program by January 1970 may no longer receive federal funds for medical care under the public assistance programs.

In states electing to implement the new program, all persons on public assistance (federally aided categories) are to be included. The same program of services is to be made available to all persons included in the program, except that states electing to include aged persons in mental and tuberculosis hospitals are not required to extend the same services to persons under 65.

As a minimum, a medical assistance program must include (at least some of each of) the following:

- Inpatient hospital services
- Outpatient hospital services
- Other laboratory and x-ray services
- Skilled nursing home services
- Physicians' services

Additional services that the states may make available are:

- Medical care furnished by licensed practitioners
- Home health care services
- Private duty nursing services
- Clinic services
- Dental services
- Physical therapy and related services
- Prescribed drugs, dentures, prosthetic devices, and eyeglasses
- Other diagnostic, screening, preventive, and rehabilitation services
- Inpatient hospital and skilled nursing home services for individuals 65 or over in tuberculosis or mental hospitals
- Any other medical care recognized under state law.

The states are required to show progress toward broadening the scope of services available and liberalizing the (state's) eligibility requirements for medical assistance with a view toward furnishing, by July 1, 1975, comprehensive services to substantially all individuals meeting the state's eligibility standards with regard to income and resources.

No durational residence requirements may be imposed nor any lien against a recipient's property during his or her lifetime, or lifetime of spouse and surviving minor children. Financial responsibility of relatives other than for spouse or minor children may not be taken into account for purposes of determining eligibility.

Payment for inpatient hospital services is to be made on the basis of *reasonable cost*.

A single state agency is to be designated to administer the medical assistance program except that the determination of eligibility shall be made by the agency administering the program for *old age assistance* (in effect, the state's Department of Public Welfare).

Title V, Maternal and Child Health and Crippled Children's Services

- Increased grant funds are authorized for maternal and child health and crippled children's services.

- Grants are authorized for training professional personnel for care of crippled children, particularly children with multiple handicaps.

- Special Project Grants for Health of School and Preschool Children.

Grants are authorized for "projects of a comprehensive nature for health care and services for *children and youth* of school age or for pre-school children" particularly in areas with concentrations of low income families.

Grants may be made to a state or local health agency, the agency administering the Title V programs, to any school of medicine (with appropriate participation by a school of dentistry), or to any affiliated teaching hospital.

Projects are to include at least such screening, diagnosis, preventive services, treatment, correction of defects, and aftercare, both medical and dental, as may be provided for in regulations of the Secretary.

Treatment, correction of defects, or aftercare provided under the project is to be available only to children who would not otherwise receive it because they are from low income families or for other reasons beyond their control.

- Payments for inpatient hospital services are to be made on the basis of *reasonable costs.*
- Increased grant funds are authorized for child welfare services.

INDEX